Managing

Stress

in Emergency Medical Services

American Academy of Orthopaedic Surgeons

Author:

Brian Luke Seaward, Ph.D.

JONES AND BARTLETT PUBLISHERS

Sudbury, Massachusetts

BOSTON   TORONTO   LONDON   SINGAPORE

American Academy of Orthopaedic Surgeons

 Jones and Bartlett Publishers, Inc.

World Headquarters
Jones and Bartlett Publishers
40 Tall Pine Drive
Sudbury, MA 01776
978-443-5000
info@jbpub.com
www.jbpub.com

Jones and Bartlett Publishers International
Barb House, Barb Mews
London W6 7PA
UK

ISBN: 0-7637-1008-3
ISBN: 0-7637-1244-2 with audio CD

Library of Congress Cataloging-in-Publication Data

Seaward, Brian Luke.
  Managing Stress in Emergency Medical Services / Brian Luke Seaward.
    p. cm.
  ISBN 0-7637-1008-3 (softcover)
  ISBN 0-7637-1244-2 (with audio CD)
  1. Emergency medical personnel—Job stress.   2. Stress management.
  3. Emergency medical personnel—Mental health.   4. Emergency medical
services.   I. Title.
RA645.5.S43   2000
362.18—dc21
                                                    99-29196
                                                      CIP

Senior Acquisitions Editor: Tracy Foss
Associate Editor: Caroline Fitzpatrick
Director of Design and Production: Anne Spencer
Senior Production Editor: Cynthia Knowles Maciel
Manufacturing Director: Therese Bräuer
Manufacturing Buyer: Kristen Guevara
Design and Composition: Studio Montage
Cover Photograph: ©Phillip Wallick, The Stock Market
Printing and Binding: Banta Company

Additional credits appear on page 84 which constitutes a continuation of the copyright page.
Printed in the United States of America
03 02 01 00 99   10 9 8 7 6 5 4 3 2 1

Contents

Chapter 3: Effective Coping Skills 30

Acknowledgements

Special thanks go to my assistant Susan Griffin, to my colleague Jay Bradshaw, State of Maine EMS, and to the wonderful staff at Jones and Bartlett who assisted in this project: Caroline Fitzpatrick, Cynthia Knowles Maciel, Tracy Foss, and Mike DeFronzo.

We would like to thank the following people for their invaluable reviews:

Sarah A. Bohn, Ph. D
Clinical Psychologist
Carlsbad, California

Robert Carter, NREMT-P
Paramedic, Baltimore City Fire Department
Instructor, EMS Training Committee
Clinical Associate, Pediatric Intensive Care Unit
The Johns Hopkins Children's Center
Baltimore, Maryland

Linda Frissora-Gosselin, REMT, IC
Quinsigamond Community College
Millbury, Massachusetts

Carol Gupton, BSEMS, NREMT-P
EMS Faculty, Training Division
Omaha Fire Department
Omaha, Nebraska

Gregg S. Margolis, MS, NREMT-P
Assistant Professor, University of Pittsburgh
Associate Director of Education, Center for Emergency Medicine
Pittsburgh, Pennsylvania

Jose Salazar, MPH, NREMT-P
President, Jose Salazar & Associates
Sterling, Virginia
Training Officer, Loudon County CISM Team
Loudon, Virginia

Mike Taigman, EMT-P
Co-Owner, Sempai-Do L.L.C.
Oakland, California

Walk-Through

www.StressLessEMS.com

www.StressLessEMS.com

Web links, which are found throughout each chapter, indicate that more information can be found on that subject on the Internet. Simply go to www.StressLessEMS.com, select the appropriate chapter, and choose the link. These links provide constantly updated information on some of the most important concepts in the book.

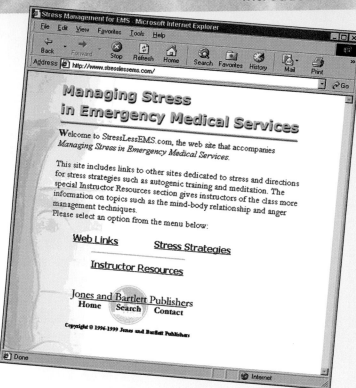

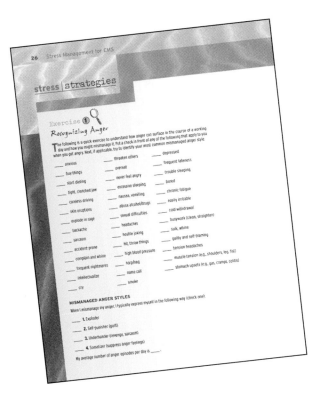

Stress Strategies

These end-of-chapter activities provide a way for students to practice the concepts learned in the chapter. Students will have a chance to learn how to both mentally and physically relax, from recording their dreams to doing autogenic training. Space has been provided for students to finish the activities in this book. All Stress Strategies should be considered confidential.

Additional Resources

Instructor's Toolkit for Managing Stress in Emergency Medical Services: This CD-ROM offers PowerPoint slide show presentations that allow you to glide through the presentation with ease, as well as customizable lesson plans. ISBN: 0-7637-1052-0

Instructor's Manual: These detailed lesson plans and teaching tips will cut your preparation time in half! ISBN: 0-7637-1050-4

Managing Stress in Emergency Medical Services Book and Relaxation CD: A relaxation audio CD is packaged with the book to offer an ideal way to practice relaxation techniques at home, in the office, or elsewhere. ISBN: 0-7637-1244-2

Chapter | I   The Stress of EMS

When Tom started as an EMT, he was told there would be stressful days, but no one told him how to deal with the stress.

As a paramedic, Julie has a sense of calmness about her, but lately, she's been bothered by intense migraines. Paul admits that he gets easily annoyed by his chatty partner and bureaucratic red tape. Dave has been a state trooper for five years, and that's about how long he has been grinding his teeth at night. Bill lost his partner and best friend while fighting a house fire, and six months later the tragic loss is still devastating. Sarah thrives on the adrenaline rush of excitement, which makes her job as a Rocky Mountain Rescue crew team member ideal, but she admits that at times, the excitement takes its toll on her physical well-being. While Kevin worries that his unit is not prepared for an episode of anthrax, Stan gets stressed just thinking about the low pay for the amount of work and overtime he puts in. These and other stories are not uncommon among the professionals who constitute the working force of Emergency Medical Services. If there is a common thread among these stories, it is that the undercurrent of stress is ever present for people who serve in the role of assisting others in need.

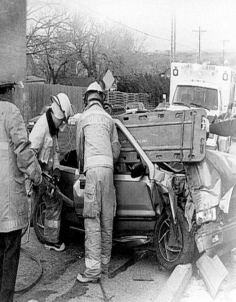

Every emergency professional needs to have excellent stress management skills.

Rocky Mountain Rescue Team Member

Today, the boundaries between professional duties and personal life are extremely thin and very permeable. On-the-job stress can easily spill over into your personal life and affect your health, your relationships, and your mental well-being. Stress, the "equal opportunity destroyer," affects everyone regardless of gender, career, income, or geographic location. Typical occupational stressors include personality conflicts, excessive meetings, voluminous reports, tight deadlines, and budget constraints; but as an Emergency Medical Services (EMS) professional, you must also deal with poor advancement opportunities, citizens with scanners, news reporters, language barriers with non-native English speakers, and too many fund-raisers, not to mention the occupational hazards of mass casualty incidents. You need to make stress management a priority, so neither your job performance nor your personal integrity is compromised and your personal life doesn't suffer. As you read this workbook, keep in mind that you deal with two levels of occupational stress: the basic day-to-day work dynamics and the high-performance tasks of patient care.

By its very nature, your work as an EMS professional—providing high-quality patient care—is stressful. Additional stress factors include interrupted family gatherings, boring long-distant transports, and the feeling of being under the microscope of both the media and living room armchair EMTs. Although only a small percentage of calls involve crises, trauma, accidents, or life-threatening situations, when these occur, they intensify your physical stress. The average person rarely encounters these situations. But for you, an EMS professional, they constitute a critical aspect of your job description and carry inherent potential stress-related issues.

In earlier periods of human history, the major stress was to ensure physical survival. For the average person today, stress involves more mental, emotional, and/or spiritual issues. The role of many EMS professionals (particularly police and fire rescue, paramedics, and rescue teams) can often put them physically at risk, yet requires them to maintain a sense of calm and level-headedness under a cloud of potential panic. Even EMS staff members behind the scenes at the station must be poised, ready, alert, and quick to respond at some level. Eventually, this pressure takes its toll on all aspects of your well-being, making you more vulnerable to the long-term consequences of stress. For this reason, essential stress management skills are crucial for high-quality performance, regardless of the type of stressor involved or what role you play in emergency assistance and patient care.

Good stress management skills are life skills. Because EMS professionals in the field have a higher risk of occupational stress than the average person, this book is designed specifically to help you constantly refine stress management skills so that you can live your life with a greater sense of balance. However, these same stress management skills are also essential life skills for all levels of support staff within the realm of EMS. The purpose of this workbook is to provide you with the essential skills necessary to cope with a host of occupational stressors, from routine duties to high-risk performance. As you read through this workbook, regardless of what examples are given, think about how you can best apply the information throughout all aspects of your life.

> **Essential stress management skills are crucial for high-quality performance, regardless of the type of stressor involved or what role the person plays in emergency assistance and patient care.**

A Closer Look at Stress

www.StressLessEMS.com

Researchers agree that stress is best defined as a "perceived threat." Regardless of the stressor (whether real or imagined), all threats cascade from mind to body, resulting in a rush of stress hormones (epinephrine, norepinephrine, cortisol, aldosterone) and urging the body into some state of physical readiness. This is the first stage of the general adaptation syndrome. The stress hormones produce an increase in heart rate, blood pressure, ventilation, muscle tension, and metabolism, preparing the body to fight or flee. For the most part, on-the-job stressors that you may encounter, such as morbidly obese patients, antiquated equipment, or restrictive bureaucratic policies, are not a threat to your physical existence. However, police, firefighters, and paramedic rescuers on the front lines of EMS must constantly be on the alert and physically ready for action. Back at the station or in your private life, these perceived threats can have a more mental (overwhelmed with tasks), emotional (unresolved anger or fear), or spiritual (questioning relationships, values, and purpose in life) nature. Therefore, the best approach to learn effective stress management skills is twofold: first, recognize the factors of occupational stress (and maintain a sense of calm) in both professional and personal situations; and second, employ effective stress management skills in an effort to resolve the issues when stress arises.

The focus of this book is holistic, dealing with both mind (causes of stress) and body (symptoms of stress). The material is organized to help you deal with the causes of stress using effective mental coping techniques (reframing, humor, time management, communication skills, journal writing, and creative problem solving). You can also learn how to deal with the symptoms of stress (muscle tension, insomnia, illness) using effective physical relaxation techniques (physical exercise, meditation, mental imagery, autogenic training, yoga, and t'ai chi). The overriding purpose of a holistic stress management program is to give you

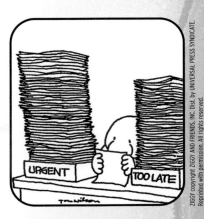

Worksite stress often results from feeling overwhelmed with responsibilities.

the skills you will need to regain and/or maintain a sense of physical and mental homeostasis. By integrating the use of effective coping skills and relaxation techniques in your professional and your personal life, you will have a more balanced and healthy life. It is essential that you, as a health care professional working in the field of patient care and emergency assistance, take as good care of yourself as you do those whom you help. No one else is going to do it for you. Additionally, not only will these techniques serve you, but once you become proficient, you may be able to share some of these skills with the people receiving emergency assistance.

Optimal Stress Curve

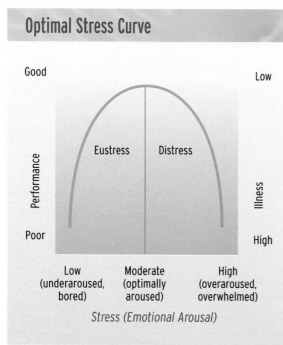

The Yerkes-Davidson Curve illustrates that, to a point, stress or arousal can actually increase performance. Stress to the left of the midpoint is considered to be eustress (good). Stress beyond the midpoint, however, is believed to detract from performance and/or health status and is therefore labeled distress (bad).

Good Stress and Bad Stress

Virtually any experience, situation, memory, or thought can promote stress—from encountering a spider or snake for the first time to merely thinking about missing a bus. In simple terms, stress can be categorized in two ways: good stress and bad stress. Good stress, or eustress, is any type of stimulation that is inspiring or motivating. Examples might include being promoted, receiving an award, or accomplishing a challenging goal. Good stress is rarely the topic of everyday conversation, nor is it addressed in newspaper articles or television headlines. But it's fair to say that you, as an EMS professional, will often encounter this type of stress. In fact, most rescue professionals in the field say that this type of stress is necessary to get the job done and done well; it sparks the surge of adrenaline that accompanies the first responder's call.

Bad stress is often called "distress" or just plain "stress." The continuum of distress ranges from complete boredom (sitting around agitated, waiting and waiting for a call, with no stimulus to engage you) to "sensory overload," or feeling completely overwhelmed and incapable of dealing with the problem(s) at hand. (Imagine a dispatcher flooded with a hundred disaster calls or a small town unit of four dealing with an airplane crash.) The optimal amount of stress lies somewhere between these two extremes. The optimal point varies from person to person, making a one-size-fits-all stress management program impossible to design. Moreover, this optimal stress level varies from day to day and from experience to experience for each individual. For this reason, it is imperative that you become aware of your daily stress levels and use the skills that work for you so that you can maintain your optimal stress level. The optimal stress curve illustration shows that there is a fine balance between too little and too much stress. Too little stress can lead to boredom, while too much stress can result in feelings of being completely overwhelmed and stressed out.

Stress comes in two forms: acute and chronic, or cumulative. As you read the description of these two forms of stress, think of examples in your life that fall into these categories.

Acute Stress

Acute stress surfaces quickly, is extremely intense, and tends to run its course in a short period of time (usually less than 5 to 30 minutes). Arriving at the scene of a serious car accident or multiple drowning and entering a burning building are examples of acute stress. The average person might encounter acute stress once a month. The same cannot be said for you, the EMS professional (particularly field providers). On average, you are more likely to encounter one to several episodes per week, depending on where you live. The state of repeated physical arousal can dull your mental acuity and become a real drain on your physical and emotional energy.

Add to these examples acute stress from interactions with peers, supervisors, or medical staff; car problems; phone tag; traffic to and from work, and it is easy to see that acute stress plays a significant role in the total stress picture. Acute stress can be a double-edged sword, for it provides the adrenaline rush of excitement that many thrive on. However, the repeated surge of stress hormones in the course of a day not only heightens the threshold for more excitement, it also lowers the resistance to the physical wear-and-tear process of the body's stress general adaptation syndrome, as described by famed stress researcher Hans Selye. This is why stress management techniques are so important: to maintain a sense of equilibrium in the course of each day.

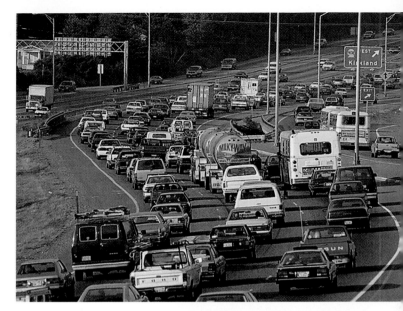

Chronic Stress

Chronic stress (cumulative stress) is not as intense as acute stress in the immediate effect it has on heart rate and blood pressure, yet this type of stress can linger for weeks, months, years, and even decades. Personality conflicts, irritating work conditions, repeated overtime hours, family strife, recurring financial difficulty, prolonged grief, job burnout, and unresolved marital issues all qualify as chronic stressors. Two classic examples cited by EMS professionals are frustrating work-family dynamics and grief over the death of a colleague. As the stress from one or more of these issues continues, it can not only exacerbate worksite issues, it can also invade your personal life—physically, mentally, emotionally, and spiritually.

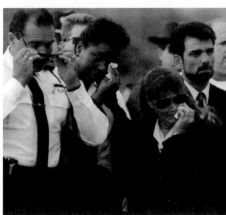

Stressors can be either short-term, such as being caught in traffic, or long-term, such as grieving the loss of a family member. It is the long-term stressors that seem to have the greatest consequence on our health.

The feelings resulting from cumulative stress are often expressed in daily emotions such as impatience, frustration, a short attention span, hostility, depression, doubt, anxiety, guilt, worry, or apathy. At the work site, these feelings can also show up as pessimism, inability to focus, job dissatisfaction, job burnout, sarcasm, or absenteeism. If you are experiencing chronic stress, you can put yourself, other squad members, and your patient at risk (90% of accidents are the result of human error caused by problems such as a wandering mind). Data compiled by several researchers, including Ken Pelletier and Candace Pert, reveal that long-term unresolved stress will ultimately have a detrimental effect on your physical health, causing a range of illnesses from the common cold to cancer. (Stress and disease is discussed in more depth in Chapter 2.)

The Stress Response

www.StressLessEMS.com

The phrase "fight or flight response" was coined by Harvard physiologist Walter Cannon around 1932 to describe the dynamics involved in the body's survival response to physical danger. Perhaps it is no surprise that it's this same energy system that EMS professionals use in the field when responding to an emergency situation, whether it is a natural disaster, a terrorist attack, or a mass casualty incident. It is also the identical energy system (with less intensity) that is used when you avoid a pending issue or when you confront a co-worker or a medical staff member with whom you are having problems. Under stress, the body prepares itself for

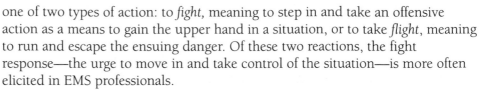

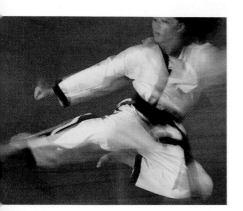

one of two types of action: to *fight,* meaning to step in and take an offensive action as a means to gain the upper hand in a situation, or to take *flight,* meaning to run and escape the ensuing danger. Of these two reactions, the fight response—the urge to move in and take control of the situation—is more often elicited in EMS professionals.

As described by Daniel Goleman in his book *Emotional Intelligence,* the fight response is rooted in *anger.* In professional athletics, the term used to describe this response is "controlled aggression" as athletes channel their stress energy (primarily anger) to overcome their physical challenge. Conversely, the flight response is initiated by *fear.* Both anger and fear are strong motivating factors for performance, and EMS professionals on the front lines of crisis call on the energy from both emotions in every high-risk task.

Sports psychology research has shown that Eastern European athletes are renowned for their use of controlled aggression in sporting events. EMS patient care providers (particularly police, firefighters, and paramedics) and superior athletes have much in common in this regard, because the physiologic reactions in athletic competition are identical to those experienced in emergency situations. These physiologic changes, which take place during the stress response, include increased heart rate, increased respiration, increased sweating response, increased muscle tension, and increased metabolism, all of which occur at the same time to allow for maximum performance. The response that you experience as you enter into the scene of a fire, car accident, terrorist situation, or domestic violence is identical to that experienced by an Olympic athlete in competition.

The stress response also involves converting feelings of fear into courage as the rescue is executed or emergency assistance is provided. For example, controlled aggression is elicited to step in and take control, whereas fear may be consciously (or unconsciously) present as you race against the clock to bring someone back to safety. To a much lesser extent, but of no less importance, this same response occurs in confronting squad members, bureaucratic health agencies, budget concerns, average drivers on the highway, or frustrating dynamics at the station. Control is paramount in these situations as well. Unfortunately, more often than not, our emotions, particularly fear, control us and perpetuate the stress response. A closer look at fear can help to see how these feelings, when they surface, can be addressed, resolved, and converted into the courage to act. (Anger is highlighted in Chapter 2.)

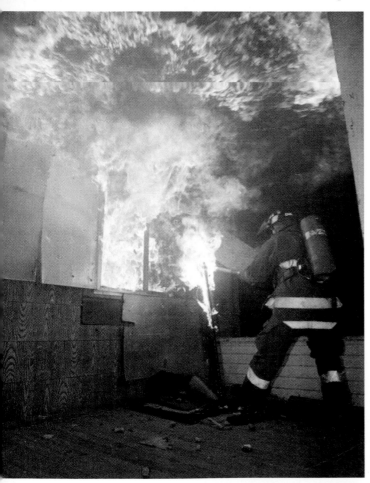

For both athletes and EMS professionals, the fight or flight response can be useful in overcoming physical challenges.

Fear: The Flight Response

Fear can impede anyone's performance, whether you are a suicide prevention counselor, a ski patroller, a water safety instructor, or an EMT arriving as a first responder to an accident. Fear can surface in many ways, from doubt to paranoia. Left unaddressed, fear can become immobilizing. The initial response to fear is avoidance, and while this may be helpful in terms of physical threats, it is ineffective with nonphysical threats. Although job responsibilities vary within the ranks of EMS professionals, consider the examples of a field commander's responsibilities during an anthrax attack. Examine how fear can surface in several ways in this situation and in your own line of work. In an effort to ensure the safety of the rescue unit, as well as those affected by the threat, the fear of this first-time encounter could inhibit his or her performance to give commands properly.

Fear of Failure

The fear of failure is based on how you perceive your own thoughts and actions, such as when you do not feel you achieved success with a task (e.g., conducting a Critical Incident Stress Debriefing (CISD) session or a first time on-camera interview). Fear of failure is particularly common for EMS professionals who are new to the field and is often associated with feelings of guilt. The best way to deal with the fear of failure is to acknowledge your strengths, realize that there are some things that are beyond your control, and, perhaps most important, understand that failure may sometimes be not the lack of accomplishment, but rather the lack of effort involved with a task.

Fear of Rejection

Fear of rejection is like the fear of failure, but this fear is based on your perception of how others will perceive or judge your performance, whereas fear of failure is your judging of yourself. It is not uncommon for EMS professionals to fear rejection from colleagues, supervisors, or families of those involved with accidents. The best way to deal with the fear of rejection is to accept that you are not your job, and to know that your self-worth is not based solely on your career. (Self-esteem building is addressed in Chapter 2.) Second, know that comments and feedback from other people in the midst of crisis may be rooted in their own fears, which they then project (as an ego defense mechanism) onto you. You should not take on other people's emotional baggage. Positive self-feedback is a good habit to employ on and off the job to combat fear of rejection. (This skill is addressed in more detail in Chapter 2.)

Fear of the Unknown

Fear of the unknown is a common fear in situations where information is in short supply. Unfamiliarity can lead to uncertainty and doubt, and these in turn can affect your performance. Ways to deal with fear of the unknown include gathering information; relying on what information you do know and what skills you have; faith; and using a synthesis of instinct, intuition, and collective wisdom from your previous experiences (which may be all you have to go on) to get you through this new situation.

Fear of Death and Dying

Fear of death and dying is said to be the "mother of all fears." Fear of death and dying is a universal fear, and to a large extent, fear of the unknown is involved as well. Because most people today are shielded from many aspects of the death and dying process, this mysterious aspect augments the fear factor. Fear of death and dying also involves the fear of pain and raises issues of spiritual well-being (relationships, aspects of values, and purpose in life). Inner resources such as faith, compassion, humbleness, forgiveness, courage, and patience are cited as means to manage the stress elicited by fear of death and dying. Because you deal with death and dying regularly, often under grim circumstances, coping skills, particularly black or gallows humor, can help you diffuse the fear factor. (Coping skills are addressed in more detail in Chapter 3.)

> Inner resources such as faith, compassion, humility, forgiveness, courage, and patience are ways to manage stress.

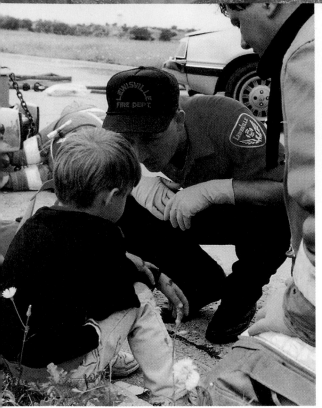

You can share the coping skills you will learn in this book with your patients to help them deal with the stress of being injured.

Use the Fight or Flight Response for Its Intended Purpose

It is important to state again that the fight or flight response is a survival dynamic that the body uses when confronted by physical threats. While this is an appropriate response for emergency assistance, it is an inappropriate (or at least antiquated) response for nonphysical threats, such as personality conflicts, a lack of state-of-the-art equipment, frustrations with other staff members, and run-ins with various agencies. The constant flood of stress hormones released into the bloodstream and the increased metabolic activity to various target organs can eventually lead to serious long-term health problems. (The negative impact of stress is discussed in Chapter 2.) The expression "respond rather than react" is as appropriate for dealing with personal stressors of a psychologic nature at the station as it is for giving emergency assistance, when you need to keep your wits about you.

The Role of the Ego

The purpose of the ego is to protect the self from harm when danger is present or a perceived threat is near. The ego does this in a number of ways, which Sigmund Freud referred to as "defense mechanisms," including denial ("This isn't happening"), rationalization ("It's okay because everyone does it"), repression ("I don't remember that happening"), or projection ("You made me hit you"). Freud's theory that defense mechanisms are used to shield the self from emotional and even physical pain is commonly accepted. Typically, several defense mechanisms are used in combination, and the bigger the danger, the greater the extent to which they are employed. When it comes to stress, the ego is always present, although it's not necessarily the bad guy (unless it dominates all behavior). The ego is used for survival, because it activates the fight or flight response. This response is good (in moderate amounts) when you are in physical danger or when quick decisions are essential, but it can be extremely unproductive for nonphysical threats. In fact, using defense mechanisms with nonphysical stressors can actually perpetuate the stress response.

It is not uncommon for EMS professionals to employ these defense mechanisms in the line of duty. After the emergency rescue is complete, however, there needs to be time to process the event so that thoughts and feelings can be quickly resolved rather than be allowed to lie dormant. Unless some resolution is reached, these thoughts and feelings can result in latent emotional distress or contribute toward post-traumatic stress disorder (PTSD). (PTSD is explained further in Chapter 2.) This is the reason for CISD: to diffuse the emotional distress from an acute incident, as described below.

CISD will help you deal with emotionally draining incidents.

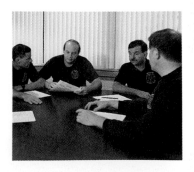

Critical Incident Stress Debriefing

www.StressLessEMS.com

In the EMS profession, the epitome of acute stress is felt during what are commonly known as "critical incidents." These emergencies are intense and can be physically and emotionally draining. Because of the nature of the stress involved in critical incidents, a special protocol of stress intervention has been designed defining the parameters of a critical incident. The following review of CISD is adapted from the work of Jeffrey T. Mitchell and the Holeman Group.

CISD Dynamics During an Incident

The first aspect of CISD involves both on-scene support services and defusing stress immediately following the event. A debriefing team provides on-scene support services to assist obviously distressed personnel. Defusings are described as "short unstructured debriefings" to reduce acute stress by discussing the details of the event. This session is typically conducted upon return to the station and is short (about 30 to 60 minutes). Demobilizations, like defusings, take place immediately after an incident, particularly a large-scale incident; however, in contrast to the defusing or debriefing, personnel are not obligated to discuss the incident. Talking is optional in this half-hour session, after which all personnel are encouraged to rest either at the station or at home before resuming their routine duties.

CISD Dynamics After an Incident

Because emotional reactions can be so intense in the first 24 hours after a critical incident, a formal CISD is typically scheduled by a CISD team several days after the critical incident. A formal CISD is both a psychological and educational support group discussion under the guidance of a well-prepared CISD team. The purpose of CISD is to enable personnel to return to their routine lives as quickly as possible. This procedure has seven phases.

First, a formal CISD is initiated with an introduction by the CISD team members. Personnel are reminded that all material is confidential. Second, facts of the incident are discussed as staff members describe in their own words what happened at the scene. Third, the debriefing team leader initiates a discussion called a *thought phase* to help staff members to personalize their experience. Rather than facts, they describe how they personally experienced the event. The fourth phase is called the *reaction phase,* in which personnel share what they consider to be the worst part of the event. It is this phase that is most cathartic in dealing with emotions triggered by the incident. The *symptom phase* is the fifth step in the process, in which the team leader asks personnel to identify stress symptoms at three distinct times: initially during the incident, three to five days after the incident, and later. The symptom phase is followed by the *teaching phase,* in which group members are taught several stress management techniques (like those in this workbook) as well as grief processing and communication skills that can be used with spouses and significant support group members. The last phase is the *reentry phase,* in which group members are given a chance to ask questions. After any discussion, the CISD is concluded. At this time, if the CISD team members feel that one or more of the participants might benefit from counseling, referrals are made.

> Let there be no doubt; burnout is a very real phenomenon in EMS.

Let's Talk About Burnout

· ·

It is quite common in all service-related careers to experience burnout from the day-to-day experience of caregiving. In this regard, EMS professionals are no different than other public service professionals such as physicians, nurses, or schoolteachers, who also experience high levels of burnout. Burnout is a very real phenomenon in EMS. The emotional demands of the job, the expectation of additional work hours, extended shifts, overtime, and the lack of appreciation all contribute to feelings of burnout. When personal and family responsibilities are added to the mix, the word "burnout" barely begins to describe the feelings of mental, emotional, and physical exhaustion. Just thinking about going to work can be energy draining and even nauseating. The result affects not only you personally, in terms of attitude, personality, and quality of work, but also the people you attend to as a professional caregiver. The purpose of an effective stress management program is to provide the opportunity for regaining balance, giving you a chance to recharge your personal energy source so that the incidence and feelings of burnout are greatly minimized.

Occupational stressors vary from job to job (e.g., from dispatcher to paramedic). However, there are some common issues that frequently arise. Additionally, each career position (e.g., squad commander, police officer, firefighter) has stressors that are specific to one's work conditions as well. Moreover, paid providers have different stressors than those of volunteers. What are common stressors for individuals who are involved with EMS? Although stressors vary from one person to the next, the following is a short list divided into two categories: occupational stressors and personal stressors. Check this list and see whether you can relate or identify with any of these common stressors. Becoming aware of these issues is the first step in resolving them. Complete Exercise 1 to make your own list of occupational and personal stressors.

Stress may be a fact of life, but it doesn't have to rule your life. Stress can be perceived as both good and bad, but the most damaging stress is that which is left unresolved. Take a good look at those issues which promote stress in your life and learn to resolve them quickly.

 F o r   Y o u r   I n f o r m a t i o n

Occupational Stressors

- Long or extended shifts
- Value conflicts (dealing with minorities, immigrants, people of different religions or sexual orientations, etc.)
- Management conflicts
- Poor advancement opportunities
- Poor system designs
- Problems with supervisors
- Problems with instructors or physicians
- Incompetent partners, poor peer support
- Bureaucratic (agency) conflicts

- Little recognition
- Job burnout
- Expectations of the public
- Life and death issues
- Poor pay or other compensation
- Hazardous work conditions
- Mass casualty incidents
- Threats of terrorism
- Dealing with the media
- Overeager citizens with police scanners
- Fear of inadequate training or not enough training

- Poor professional communication skills
- Not enough action
- Too many charity events—pancake breakfasts, bean suppers, and car washes
- Obstructive people
- Too much overtime
- Insufficient budget for equipment upgrades
- Having to stay emotionally neutral in dealing with victims and perpetrators

Personal Stressors

- Lack of high-quality family time
- Lack of personal time
- Marital problems

- Financial difficulties
- Car problems, traffic
- Personal health concerns

- Others

stress | strategies

Exercise ①
Identifying Your Stressors

One of the first goals in stress management is to increase your awareness of your thoughts, feelings, and perceptions. To begin this series of workbook exercises, make a list of your top ten current stressors. Try to identify the things (both profes- sional and personal) that worry, upset, or frustrate you at the present time. List them as either occupational or personal stres- sors. *As with all of these workbook exercises, this is confidential.*

LIST *YOUR* TOP 10 STRESSORS

Occupational Stressors	Personal Stressors
FEARS	FEARS
1.	1.
2.	2.
3.	3.
4.	4.
5.	5.
FRUSTRATIONS	FRUSTRATIONS
6.	6.
7.	7.
8.	8.
9.	9.
10.	10.

PERSONAL STRESS SCALE

On a scale of 0 to 10 (0 = no stress and 10 = maximal stress/burnout), rate where you feel your personal occupational stress level is at the present time.

0	1	2	3	4	5	6	7	8	9	10
I	I	I	I	I	I	I	I	I	I	I

Exercise ②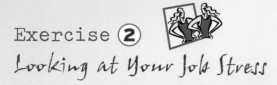

Looking at Your Job Stress

The following personal and confidential assessment is adapted from the American Institute of Stress. It is designed to help you determine your own level of workplace stress. Please take a few minutes to rank each of the 10 questions on a sliding scale from 1 to 10, as shown. Then total your score and decide whether you agree with the results.

   1 = strongly disagree with the statement

   5 = neither agree nor disagree with the statement

  10 = strongly agree with the statement

WORK STRESS SURVEY

_____ **1.** At work, I can't say what I really think or get things off my chest.

_____ **2.** My job has a lot of responsibilities, but I don't have much authority or autonomy (or I have too much).

_____ **3.** I tend to spend more time at work than I would like.

_____ **4.** I seldom receive adequate acknowledgment or appreciation when my work is really good or I have performed well.

_____ **5.** In general, I'm not particularly proud of my job or satisfied with my job.

_____ **6.** I don't feel that I am adequately compensated for the work I do.

_____ **7.** My workplace environment is not very pleasant or particularly safe.

_____ **8.** My job interferes with my family, social obligations and personal needs.

_____ **9.** I tend to have frequent run-ins with my supervisors, co-workers, or clients/patients or others (e.g., media personnel, ambulance chasers).

_____ **10.** Most of the time, I feel that I have little control over my life at work.

TOTAL

_____ Please add up the number you gave each question. Total your job stress score.

Legend for your job stress score:

10 – 29   = low job stress (Good job! Keep doing what you're doing!)

30 – 50   = moderate job stress (Coping skills and relaxation techniques are encouraged.)

51 – 75   = high job stress (Copings skills and relaxation techniques are encouraged.)

76 – 100 = VERY HIGH job stress (Professional counseling is recommended.)

Source: Adapted from "Reduce Job Stress Before It Reduces You," *Health and Safety,* November 1992, pages 40–43.

Negative Effects of Stress

Chapter|2

The Big Thompson Flood in Colorado occurred over twenty years ago, but to this day, Kelly still dreams of dead bodies strewn all over the canyon, particularly one image of several people trapped in a car that was washed away when the dam broke.

For Todd, the worst part of a rescue is facing the family of a patient and explaining that their loved one must be rushed to the hospital and may be in danger of losing his or her life. As a policeman, Chad delivered five babies in the past year alone, but he almost missed the arrival of his own son because he had to work overtime. It's not uncommon for Chad to feel some guilt, resentment, and frustration over trying to balance career and family.

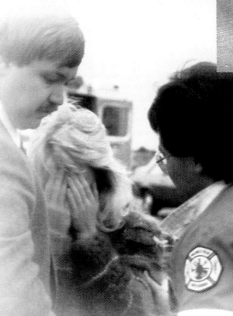

As many EMS professionals will share, their work experiences often defy description, nor are they the desired topic of everyday conversation among friends. Even after hundreds, if not thousands of encounters involving trauma and death, the humanness of each situation is never completely lost. After all, a callous heart is counterproductive to the work of a firefighter, police officer, lifeguard, dispatcher, EMT, or anyone involved in patient care. Additionally, stressful situations back at the station and in your personal life set the stage for an even stronger emotional impact, no matter what kind of personality you have.

Before examining ways to deal effectively with everyday stress, it is imperative to understand just how much of a toll stress takes on your emotional and physical well-being. First and foremost, you must realize that stress involves both mind and body and that there is no separation between the two. They are equally affected. Unresolved emotional stress (whether it be the boredom of a quiet 48-hour shift, the frustration of responding to repeated false alarms, or the grief of a mass casualty accident) perpetuates more feelings of stress, and physical symptoms of stress soon begin to appear. As the saying goes, "The body becomes the battlefield for the war games of the mind," meaning that all the body's physiological systems (such as the digestive, immune, or nervous systems) reflect the difficulties of a mind in turmoil. Effective stress management gently breaks the stress cycle and brings you to a greater sense of peace.

This chapter is divided into two parts. The first part deals with the emotional aspects of stress, including concerns with post-traumatic stress disorder (PTSD), grief, fatigue, anger, boredom, and low self-esteem. The second part of this chapter discusses the physical aspects of stress and how to minimize, if not avoid altogether, the physical symptoms that are so closely tied to emotions.

Thoughts become chemicals. They can kill or cure.

Bernie Siegel, MD

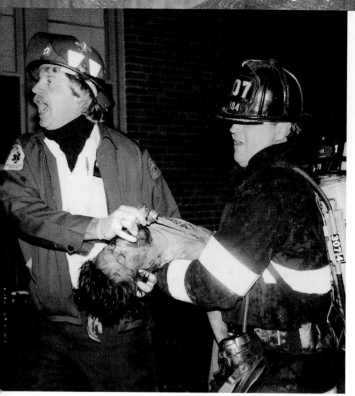

The memory of stressful events can linger in the unconscious mind, setting the stage for post-traumatic stress disorder (PTSD).

Emotional Stress

Post-Traumatic Stress Disorder

Gruesome car wrecks. Dismembered bodies. Severe burns over the entire body. Repeatedly viewing such disturbing scenes makes you vulnerable to nightmares, flashbacks, or intrusive memories that bring you back to the scene, again and again. For the purposes of stress management, trauma is best defined as a seriously distressing event that is outside the course of everyday life situations. PTSD is an emotional imbalance due to recurring memories or experiences of severe trauma. Because of the nature of your job description, you may be prone to PTSD. The most common emotional defense is *avoidance* (an ineffective coping skill for any stressor) as expressed through denial (e.g., "That wasn't really bad, I barely remember it"). Despite the denial factor or suppression (two of the ego's defense mechanisms), you may experience the effects of PTSD through memory flashbacks, dreams, or the manifestation of feelings associated with depression.

Symptoms of PTSD

People with PTSD tend to be edgy, irritable, nervously watchful, and easily startled, according to the *Harvard Medical Health Letter.* Some are fixated on trauma, while others repress or deny details of the event (also known as dissociation). As a rule, people who suffer from PTSD don't sleep very well (they have less REM dream sleep), and over the course of time, their concentration skills diminish. In some cases, there are frequent outbursts of anger and violence. Reports indicate that many people use alcohol to take the emotional edge off, which may lead to a dependency on alcohol or similar substance and result in addiction. Research indicates that the most common symptom of PTSD is depression.

Why do some people, under the same circumstances, show symptoms of PTSD while others don't? There doesn't seem to be a clear-cut answer. Experts suggest that the reason is mostly likely a combination of various exposures to trauma, specific personality types (e.g., a stress-prone versus stress-resistant or hardy personality), personality traits (such as faith, humor, or assertiveness), or biological variability (e.g., some people produce and secrete more catecholamines, or stress neurotransmitters, than others, keeping memories more current).

Post-Traumatic Stress Relief for EMS Professionals

To release memories of traumatic events, you can debrief with your co-workers about the event or keep a journal—writing not only the details of the event, but describing your thoughts and feelings on paper as a means to consciously release these memories from your mind. Art therapy lets you express thoughts, feelings, and memories through the use of pastels, crayons, or even clay, which helps create equilibrium between the conscious and unconscious minds. Frequently, the unconscious mind, which retains thoughts, feelings, and memories from these types of events, speaks a language of color, symbol, and style unlike that of the verbal and linear conscious mind. (Art therapy and journal writing are discussed further in Chapter 3.) Either art therapy, journal therapy, or both can be powerful tools for healing PTSD.

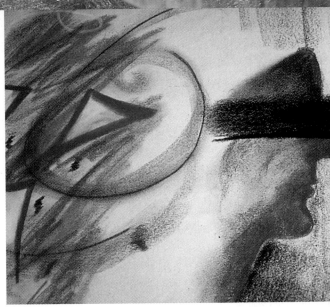

Art therapy serves as a catharsis for anger and fear.

Stages of Death and Grieving

Most of the stress people experience results from unmet expectations or, stated differently, the death of expectations, the most obvious being the death of a human being. For you, this includes mass casualty, infant and child trauma, and in particular, the loss of a co-worker. In the 1960s, Elizabeth Kübler-Ross did pioneering research on death and the grieving process. Her work has become the hallmark of psychology in this area. Although her research was with terminal cancer patients, the stages of grieving (albeit in different intensities) are identical, regardless of the perception of the stressor involved. By recognizing these stages, we can move through the grieving process at a healthier pace and not prolong the process (as many people do). As you read through these stages, reflect on any stressor in your own life involving the loss or death of an expectation.

In her most acclaimed book, *On Death and Dying,* Kübler-Ross described the following stages of the grief process. These stages have been adapted here to include two examples: the first is the death of a close colleague; the second is perhaps a more common stressor, required overtime during the weekend. Obviously, the time spent in each stage will vary from person to person. The greater the loss, the more likely that each phase will require a longer period.

1. *Denial:* Denial is a refusal to accept the truth of a situation. Denial can also manifest itself as shock. In many cases, it is a temporary rejection of the truth. With the death of a close colleague, denial begins with shock and disbelief. In the case of required overtime, the response may be, "Not again. It must be a mistake. Not this weekend!"

2. *Anger:* The anger stage can be described as a period of rage, which may include yelling, pounding, crying, and/or deep frustration manifesting in a physical-emotional sense. Anger becomes a physical outlet for hostile feelings. Kübler-Ross typically saw anger directed not only at clinicians and family members, but also toward a higher power, even by people who claimed not to believe in one. In this stage, anger over the loss of a colleague may surface in many ways, from impatience to rage. Similarly, anger may surface when expectations for a free weekend are scratched because of additional overtime.

3. *Bargaining:* Kübler-Ross described this phase as a very brief but important one. Bargaining is an agreement between the conscious mind and the unconscious mind involving an exchange of offerings; it is primarily a negotiation for something more. With the loss of a partner or team member, it might involve questioning: "Why him (or her), why not me?" In the case of required overtime, bargaining might begin with the thought, "Hmm, perhaps I can switch with someone else." Or, "I'll do it this weekend, but I am out of town for the next two weekends, and I am NOT working the evening shift." Or "God, I hope it's a slow night. I'm exhausted already."

4. *Depression:* This stage is best described as a quiet or passive mood of uneasiness while at the same time feeling quite overwhelmed with thoughts and responsibilities. With depression, there is very little, if any, perceived hope. With the loss of a friend, you may notice a period of emotional withdrawal and low motivation. Energy may be replaced by some level of apathy. In the case of required overtime, once the reality sets in, withdrawal may come in the form of silence, sarcasm, or similar behaviors.

> Over half the stress you experience is the result of unmet expectations.

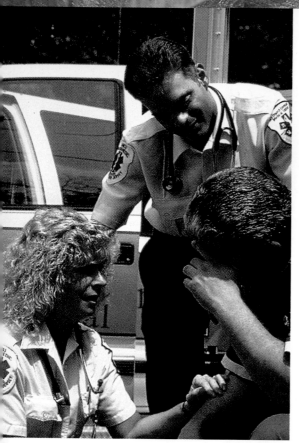

The loss of a partner can be an extremely traumatic experience.

5. *Acceptance:* If and when all previous stages of the grieving process are complete, then and only then will you arrive at the final stage of acceptance. Acceptance is an approval of the existing conditions, a receptivity to the things that cannot be changed. Acceptance is *not* giving in or giving up. It is not a surrender to the circumstances. Rather, it is a recognition of the particular situation in which you find yourself. Acceptance allows you to move on with your life. With acceptance comes hope, then faith. At this stage, there is recognition that things are better, not worse, and life goes on. In the example of extended overtime, you might say, "OK, someone's got to do it. Let's pitch in and make a good time of it." In the death of a colleague, you may come to a personal understanding about death such as, "John may have passed away, but he is still with me in spirit and I can go on."

In the acceptance stage, there is no trace of anger or pity. Kübler-Ross indicates that this stage is very difficult to arrive at, and many people don't reach it in the course of their grieving. The process of acceptance, of resolving pent-up feelings or frustrations, is not an easy one. In fact, it can be quite emotionally painful. In her work, Kübler-Ross observed some people with a stubborn streak who would rather leave matters unresolved than face this process. Still others are unsure how best to resolve these emotions and eventually become hostages to their conscious and unconscious feelings.

You can go through these stages of grieving hundreds of times in your lifetime. Considering the rate of change in today's world, these same stages of death and dying can be experienced daily. Because episodes of stress (both acute and chronic) involve unmet expectations, it's not unrealistic to experience some aspect of grieving frequently. The stress associated with the stages of death is, as Kübler-Ross explains, a catalyst to provide a greater mental awareness of several or all unresolved emotions. As you pass from one stage to the next, you enter a deeper level of mental awareness and resolution. In recent years, Kübler-Ross has amended her original concept to suggest that in some cases, one of the first four stages may even be skipped and that there may be frequent backsliding to other stages. She noted that the last stage is the most difficult to arrive at and conquer, yet also the most rewarding.

General Fatigue

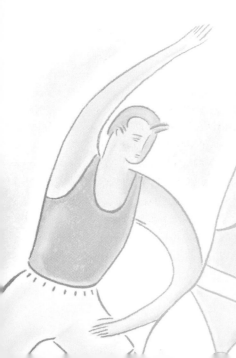

The human body is designed for periodic stress and adapts well to it. In fact, some stress, like exercise, is actually good for the body. However, the body also craves relaxation, or homeostasis. Without adequate relaxation, the body's physiology is thrown out of balance. When the body is kept in a high state of physiological arousal, specific physiological systems are taxed beyond their means, and eventually certain organs become susceptible to some level of dysfunction. Not only does repeated stress exhaust your sense of energy, but research shows that it also depletes the stores of vitamins and minerals necessary for energy production. The first sign that your body is headed in this direction is a sense of general fatigue. When fatigue sets in, the following can happen: (1) your focus on work is divided and compromised, (2) your attention span is reduced, (3) your ability to retain information is greatly limited, and (4) your decision-making process is significantly compromised. Many times, specific thoughts become magnified and distorted, making mountains out of molehills, and this too can make you feel overwhelmed both on and off the job. All of these factors can lead to mental and emotional fatigue. Over time, you can begin to lose interest in your work and become less motivated. Ultimately, both the quality of work and the quality of life suffers. More sleep doesn't necessarily mean less fatigue. Fatigue is a function of many things, including poor nutrition and mental, physical, and emotional exhaustion.

> **Fatigue is a function of many things, including poor nutrition and mental, physical, and emotional exhaustion.**

Anger and Frustration: The Fight Response

What pushes your buttons and angers or frustrates you? Generally speaking, the same things that frustrate most everyone. More specifically, a random poll elicited these answers: faulty alarms, incompetent partners, the average annoying citizen, false alarms, simple or long-distance transports, arrogant communication problems with citizens or physicians, required overtime, low pay, poor advancement opportunities, and insufficient funds for new equipment, just to name a few. These may all be valid reasons to feel frustrated, but the question is how to move beyond those issues that are beyond your control. A closer look at anger can help.

Anger is a healthy emotion, but only in minuscule amounts. First and foremost, anger is a survival emotion. Second, anger is an energizing emotion; however, anger is meant to last only seconds, supporting the adage that when you get mad, you should count to ten, then let it go. As a rule, most people don't let it go. They hang on to anger as a means of exerting some level of control, usually over

For **Y**our **I**nformation

Mismanaged Anger Styles

1. **The somatizer:** The somatizer is someone who suppresses his or her anger and rarely, if ever, shows it. As a result, anger manifests itself in the body (*soma* means "body" in Latin) as physical symptoms such as migraine headaches, hypertension, ulcers, or temporomandibular joint dysfunction. An example might be a dispatcher who never shows any frustration but has a lot of physical ailments (e.g. migraines).

2. **The self-punisher:** The self-punisher is someone who denies himself or herself a proper outlet for anger and instead substitutes for it (usually in the form of guilt) through excessive eating, sleeping, sex, exercise, or shopping.

3. **The exploder:** The exploder is someone who, when angry, erupts like a volcano and spills the emotional equivalent of hot lava in everyone's path. Road rage is a prime example. Explosive anger is expressed as a form of intimidation and is most typically used against people who will not retaliate (e.g., domestic violence).

Exploders typically make the headlines through violent acts; however, swearing and hand gestures are also characteristics of explosive behavior.

4. **The underhander:** The motto of an underhander is "Don't get mad, get even." As a form of intimidation, the underhander vents anger in what are perceived to be socially acceptable ways, such as sarcasm or showing up late for meetings, again as a control measure. An example might be a command officer manipulating a situation to make himself or herself look better for a promotion.

It should be noted that almost everyone has several of these tendencies; however, one style will typically dominate behavior. While it is good to acknowledge your anger and feel it when situations arise, it is inappropriate to mismanage anger, as the consequences are serious for everyone involved. For anger management to be effective, anger must be acknowledged and resolved quickly, not harbored indefinitely.

road to relaxation

Creative Anger Management Skills

Based on the works of Carol Tavris, Harold Weisinger, and Redford Williams and in the spirit of self-help twelve-step programs to modify unhealthy behaviors, the following suggestions are provided to help you learn to manage your anger more creatively.

1. **Know your anger style.** Is your anger style predominantly passive or active? Are you the type of person who holds anger in, or are you the kind of person who explodes? Are you a somatizer, exploder, self-punisher, or underhander? Become aware of what your current style of anger is. Take mental notes on what pushes your buttons and how you react when you get angry. Remember, recognition is the first step in changing behavior.

2. **Learn to self-monitor your anger.** Keep track of your anger in a journal or on a calendar. Write down when you get angry and what precipitates the feeling. Are there some predictable trends to your angry feelings? Ask yourself why? After you have made several entries, look for patterns of circumstances or behaviors that lead to this critical mass or boiling point of your anger.

3. **Learn to de-escalate your anger.** Rather than respond immediately, count to ten, step outside for a moment, get a drink of water, take some deep breaths, use some mental imagery to relax, and calm down. Research shows that the initial anger response is quickly followed by a long simmering process. Give yourself 10 to 20 seconds to diffuse. Take a moment to collect and regroup your mental faculties. No rational conversation can take place when someone shouts. Instead, take a time-out and remove yourself from the scene momentarily to cool off. Time-outs can help validate your feelings and give you a full perspective on the circumstance. Remember, though, that a time-out must be immediately followed by a "time-in." Find a way to let out some steam creatively and then take the next step.

4. **Learn to out-think your anger.** What are some ways to resolve this situation in a constructive way so that you and everyone involved feels better? Anger carries much energy with it. How can you best use this energy? Learn to be constructive rather than destructive.

5. **Get comfortable with all your feelings and learn to express them constructively.** People who are at most risk for stress-related diseases and illnesses are usually unable to express their feelings openly and directly. In other words, don't ignore, avoid, or repress your feelings. Anger is like a toxic acid. It needs to be treated. And it is treated by creative (constructive) expression. Try practicing the words, "I am angry!" just to verbalize your feelings. A creative approach would be to say, "I feel angry when you do..." rather than saying "I hate you when you do ..."

6. **Plan in advance.** Some situations can be identified as potential provocations of anger, and you can then create viable options to minimize your exposure to them. This is especially true of interactions with people (e.g., staff meetings, traffic, long lines at the post office). Try to plan your time wisely and work around the types of situations that are prone to light your fuse.

7. **Develop a strong support system.** Find a few close friends in whom you can confide or give vent to your frustrations. Don't force them to become allies; rather, allow them to listen and perhaps give you an insight or an objective perspective. By expressing yourself to others, you begin to process bits of information, and a clearer understanding of the situation will usually surface.

8. **Develop realistic expectations for yourself and others.** Many times anger surfaces because your expectations that you place on yourself are too high. Anger also arises when you expect too much from others such as team members, partners, and command leaders. Learn to reappraise your expectations and validate your feelings before you blow your top. Learn to reassess a situation by fine-tuning your perceptions and you will minimize anger episodes.

Continued.

9. **Learn problem-solving techniques.** Don't paint yourself into a corner without any options. Implement alternatives to situations by creating viable options to your problems. To do this, you must be willing to trust your imagination and creativity. You must also take risks with the options you have created and trust the choices you make. If your mind got you into this attitude, use your mind to get you out of it. And remember, problem-solving techniques do not include revenge or retaliation.

10. **Stay in shape.** Staying in shape means balancing your mental, emotional, physical, and spiritual well-being. Studies show that people who are in good shape bounce back from anger episodes more quickly than those who are not. Exercise is a beneficial step in the catharsis process to absolve feelings of anger. (Additional techniques are discussed in Chapter 4.) Eat good whole foods, exercise regularly, give yourself alone time or solitude, and learn to laugh more. Laughter is a great stress reducer, and gives you a better perspective on the situation at hand. Remember, though, that while laughter is the best form of medicine, anger vented in sarcasm is neither creative nor healthy for anyone.

11. **Turn complaints into requests.** Pessimists tend to complain, whine, and moan. Anyone can complain. Constant complaining indicates that you see yourself as a victim, unable to affect change. When you are frustrated with a partner, team member, or family member, rework the problem into a request for change with the person(s) involved. Seek opportunities rather than problems. Take a more optimistic outlook on how you perceive situations. This will help you frame your request.

12. **Make past anger pass.** Learn to resolve issues that have caused pain, frustration, or stress. Resolution involves an internal dialogue to work things out in your own mind and an external dialogue to resolve issues with others. Learn to forgive both yourself and others for inappropriate behavior. Forgiveness is an essential part of anger management. Set a statute of limitations on your anger and follow it.

other people. But this display of control is an illusion; instead, anger becomes the controller. This is not good for the mind, body, or spirit.

Anger shows up in a great many ways, including impatience, guilt, envy, jealousy, indignation, hostility, sarcasm, and rage. Every time you get mad, it is because of an unmet expectation (you thought your partner would show up on time and she didn't, or you thought you had a normal shift and now you're assigned overtime, or you thought there would be a backup team and there wasn't). Research shows that the average American gets angry about 15 to 20 times per day. It is important to remember that all unresolved anger becomes a control issue. But rather than gaining control, you become controlled by your anger and give your power away. Creative anger management is about resolving anger feelings and restoring a sense of personal power.

For years, anger was considered a taboo subject, even in stress management programs and books. Only fear was addressed regarding emotional stress. But what's placed on the back burner eventually boils over. Therefore, the issue of anger merits considerable attention. Today, aspects of the fight emotion are being looked at and seriously addressed. One thing is certain: people don't deal with anger very well. There are many cultural, social, and parental reasons, but in general, people tend to mismanage their anger rather than deal with it and resolve it correctly. There are four distinct styles of mismanaged anger: the somatizer, the self-punisher, the exploder, and the underhander.

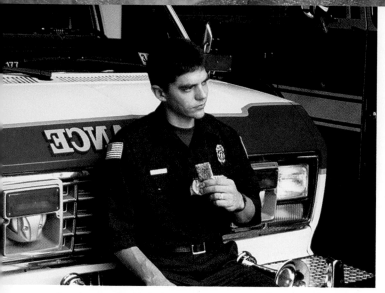

Boredom can lead to just as many problems as overstimulation does.

Boredom

Depending on where you work, EMS emergency calls fall in the categories of either feast or famine. Holidays, full moons, and natural disasters notwithstanding, calls for emergency assistance tend to be punctuated by periods of intense calm. If you just sit around and wait for the alarm to go off, the waiting game can be a bit unnerving. As one fireman stated, "Ninety percent of the time you sit around waiting for the ten percent of the time that you are called out to make a rescue." Lifeguards admit that between rescues, there are long, tedious, and monotonous periods. As one rescue worker said, "While it's nice to have a break from the action every now and then, extended periods of doing nothing can drive you nuts." Sitting around with nothing to do is boring, but so are "boring calls." These include simple transports, putting people back into bed, and other similar situations—important tasks, but without much excitement. Boredom is a combination of poor mental stimulation and poor attitude. Too little mental stimulation, just like sensory overload, can be quite stressful. In the short term, boredom can lead to potential accidents; in the long term, it challenges one's sense of self-worth and leads to low self-esteem. The basic solution to boredom is to keep your mind occupied without taxing it and to alter your (potential) negative attitude of victimization. One way to do this might include creative problem solving. (Creative problem solving is discussed in more detail in Chapter 3.)

Low Self-Esteem

High self-esteem is often described as a sense of strong self-worth and high self-acceptance. Low self-esteem is reflected in a sense of low self-worth and poor self-acceptance, always finding fault within. The things you say, the clothes you wear, and your behavior reflect your sense of self-esteem. In the North American culture, so strongly influenced by the Puritan work ethic of "worth equals work," self-esteem is often tied solely to your occupational status, work productivity, or paycheck. When occupational stress hits a critical level, your self-esteem can crumble. People with low self-esteem generate feelings of powerlessness, frustration, depression, and victimization, leading to burnout. Whereas people with low self-esteem are more susceptible to the pressures of stress, people with high self-esteem display confidence and enthusiasm and tolerate frustration well. Because a strong sense of self-esteem is critical to effective stress reduction, the primary goal in stress management programs is to help you develop and nurture high self-esteem. The four basic elements of self-esteem are connectedness, uniqueness, empowerment, and models. All of these factors need to be present and systematically cultivated throughout your life to ensure a sense of high self-esteem.

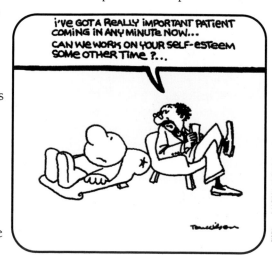

road to relaxation

Components of Self-Esteem

High self-esteem is made up of these four components:

1. **Connectedness:** A feeling of bonding and acceptance from your friends, peers, and colleagues and a sense of satisfaction that your relationships are significant and are nurtured and affirmed by others.

2. **Uniqueness:** A feeling that you have qualities that make you special and unique and that these qualities are respected and admired by others as well as by yourself.

3. **Empowerment:** A sense that you can access your inner resources to create new opportunities and use your resources and capabilities to gain and keep a sense of control in your life.

4. **Models:** Selecting people (mentors, heroes, or role models) who have certain characteristics that you would like to enhance in yourself and using these people as mentors to help you reach your highest human potential.

The following are some tips for raising your self-esteem on the job:

1. *Disarm your negative critic:* Challenge the voice inside your head that feeds put-downs and negative comments to your conscious mind. Tell yourself that you are doing a good job on the job. A critic who has only a negative side is unbalanced and dangerous to your self-esteem.

2. *Give yourself positive reinforcements and affirmations:* Remind yourself of your good qualities with truthful positive statements. Write them down, and look at the list and repeat them to yourself often in the course of a day.

3. *Avoid "should haves":* Don't place a guilt trip on yourself for unmet expectations. Learn from the past, but don't dwell on it. Look for new opportunities to grow.

4. *Focus on the qualities that make you special:* Explore your own identity and do not place all your self-worth in your job or your paycheck.

5. *Avoid comparing yourself to others:* Respect your own uniqueness and learn to cultivate it. At the same time, ask yourself who your role models are, what traits you admire in those people, and how you can foster those traits in yourself.

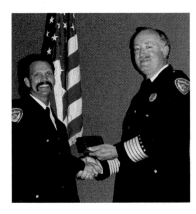

Praise from colleagues helps nurture connectedness, a pillar of high self-esteem.

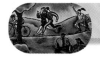

road to relaxation

Positive Affirmation Statements

1. I am calm and relaxed.
2. I have confidence in myself.
3. I am an essential member of my rescue team.
4. I am making a difference in this world.
5. I radiate success!
6. I am worthy of being respected.
7. Your positive affirmation statement:

   _____.

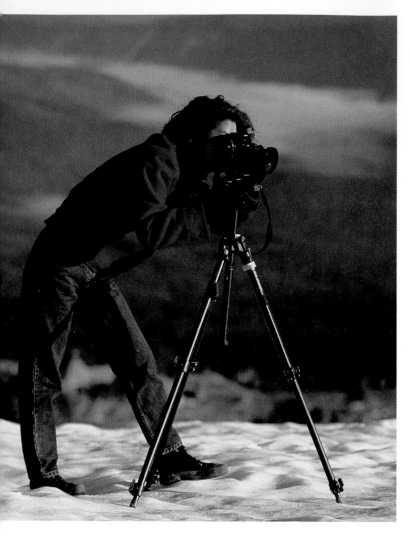

Hobbies not only serve to help build self-esteem, but actually help to nurture a sense of creativity, which often transfers back to problem- solving techniques at work.

6. *Diversify your interests:* Don't put all your eggs in one basket. Diversify your life by having many interests so that if one aspect (such as work) becomes troubled, other areas (your family or hobbies) can compensate and help you cope.

7. *Strengthen your connectedness:* Widen your network of friends inside and outside the profession. Acknowledge special places that recharge your energy, and strengthen your bonds throughout your environment. Nurture these relationships.

8. *Avoid self-victimization:* Martyrs are often admired, but begging for pity and sympathy gets old, and the effects are short lived. Don't make a habit of this; it quickly gets tiresome.

9. *Reassert yourself and your value before and during a stressful event:* Strategies used to combat stress successfully are useless unless you have a strong feeling of self-worth and self-value. Although self-esteem is abstract, it should be attended to every day, like brushing your teeth and eating. It is that important!

Physical Effects of Stress

www.StressLessEMS.com

The association between stress and disease is not a new one. For centuries physicians have suspected that emotions can significantly affect a patient's health. In the early 1970s, it was suggested that up to 50% of all disease and illness were stress-related. Recent findings about mind-body interactions estimate that up to 80% of all health-related problems are either caused or aggravated by stress. The list of such disorders is nearly endless, from the common cold to cancer, from canker soars to hemorrhoids. Clinical science has verified what was intuitive knowledge for generations: Emotions can either enhance or hinder the immune system, thereby greatly affecting your state of health.

To understand the relationship between stress and disease, it is important to know that several factors must come together to create or aggravate an illness. These include, but are not limited to, stress-promoting attitudes (unresolved anger and fear) and their effects on the nervous system, the hormonal system, and the immune system.

Research originally indicated that the repeated rush of hormones released in the fight or flight response target specific organs and cause them to dysfunction. Researchers also discovered that these same stress hormones actually destroy white blood cells, thereby lowering the body's resistance to disease and illness. Various studies now show that the human body is more complicated than was once thought. There is a direct link between emotions and the functions of white blood cells that bypasses the nervous and hormonal systems altogether. The work of people such as Norman Cousins; Bernie Siegel, M.D.; Dean Ornish, M.D.; Deepak Chopra, M.D.; Joan Borysenko, Ph.D.; Larry Dossey, M.D.; and Andrew Weil, M.D. indicate that physical health is indeed often a reflection of emotional health.

Some of the more common disorders now known to be related to the effects of chronic stress on the nervous system, the hormonal system, or the immune system are listed below. All of these illnesses have been shown to be significantly affected by a variety of relaxation techniques. (Relaxation techniques are discussed in Chapter 4.)

Aches and Pains

- *Tension headaches:* Muscle tension is the number one symptom of stress. It is most likely to appear as tension headaches, clenched jaws, stiff necks, and lower back pain. Tension headaches, the most common symptom, are produced by muscle contractions of the forehead, eyes, neck, and jaw. Most people are unaware of increased muscle tension until pain begins in the front of the head.

- *Migraine headaches:* A migraine headache is caused by an increase of blood flow and chemical secretions to the head. Symptoms can include a flash of light followed by intense throbbing, dizziness, and nausea. It is interesting to note that migraines usually do not occur in the midst of a stressor, but rather hours later. In many cases, migraines are thought to be related to an inability to express anger and frustration.

- *Temporomandibular joint dysfunction:* Repeated contraction of the jaw muscles (often during sleep) can lead to a problem called temporo-mandibular joint dysfunction (TMJ). Other symptoms include muscle pain, clicking or popping sounds when chewing, and tension headaches and earaches. Like migraines, TMJ may be associated with the inability to express feelings of anger.

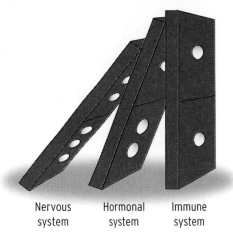

Nervous system | Hormonal system | Immune system

Three symbolic dominos representing the body's reaction to physiological stress.

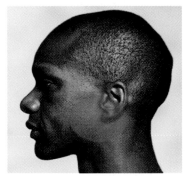

Stress can target the mandibular joint, causing temporomandibular joint dysfunction (TMJ).

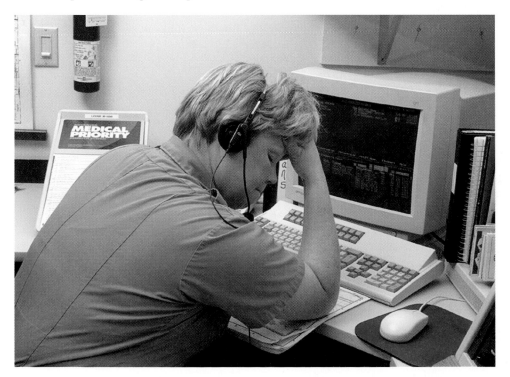

Headaches are an obvious symptom of stress.

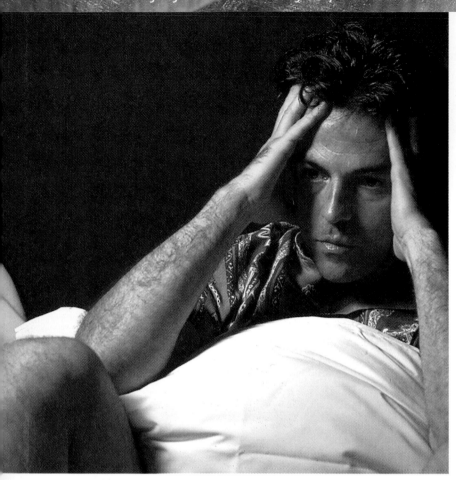

Insomnia is a common symptom
of chronic work-related stressors

Stomach Troubles

- *Ulcers and colitis:* Both the stomach and the colon are prone to ulceration and bleeding, resulting in ulcers and colitis. These conditions are not caused by foods, as once thought, but by a virus called *Helicobacter.* However, not everyone with the virus contracts ulcers, and some people get ulcers without having the virus. Stress has always been associated with ulcers, and may help create an environment conducive to the development of ulcers and colitis. Bleeding from the stomach causes nausea and vomiting. Internal bleeding from the gastrointestinal track can cause several health related problems.

- *Irritable bowel syndrome:* Irritable bowel syndrome (IBS) is characterized by repeated bouts of abdominal pain or tenderness, cramps, diarrhea, nausea, constipation, and excessive gas. Although symptoms may vary from person to person, this stress-related disorder is most commonly associated with anxiety and depression.

Nervous Anxiety

- *Insomnia:* The inability to sleep is a sure symptom of an overactive nervous system. Excessive neural stimulation to the brain and muscle tissue can cause extreme restlessness in the day or at night.

- *Bronchial asthma:* The bronchioles are tubes that carry air into the lungs. During an asthma attack, the tubes begin to fill with bronchial fluid, resulting in the person choking and gasping for air. Asthmatic attacks can be severe enough to hospitalize or kill a person and are often linked to anxiety.

- *Allergies:* An allergic reaction is initiated when a foreign substance such as a chemical, food, pollen, or dust enters the body. However, these substances are not necessary to trigger an allergic reaction. The mere memory of an attack will repeat the symptoms. It is now known that allergic reactions are more prevalent and severe when subjects are prone to anxiety. Over-the-counter medications (containing antihistamines) and allergy shots are the most common approach to dealing with allergies. Relaxation techniques are also known to minimize the effects of these foreign substances.

- *Rheumatoid arthritis:* Rheumatoid arthritis, a joint and connective tissue disease, occurs when joints swell, causing the joint tissue to become inflamed. Within time, fluid may actually enter the cartilage and bone tissue, causing further deterioration of the joint. There is speculation that rheumatoid arthritis has a genetic link as well as an association with stress. Typically, the severity of arthritic pain is related to episodes of stress, particularly to suppressed anger.

www.StressLessEMS.com

Disease and Illness

- *The common cold and influenza:* It is no coincidence that you are most likely to catch a cold when you are most stressed. When your immune defenses are down, you are more likely to succumb to nearby germs. Current findings support the idea that colds are definitely related to stress. When the immune system is suppressed, the chances of catching the flu are also greater.

- *Coronary heart disease:* Two factors link the stress response to the development of coronary heart disease. The first is high blood pressure (>145/90 mm Hg), or *hypertension.* High blood pressure is known to produce damage to the inner lining of the coronary vessels that supply the heart muscle with oxygen. The second factor involves the release of *cortisol,* which increases blood cholesterol levels, from the adrenal gland. Unfortunately, cholesterol acts as a bandage to repair damaged vessel walls, ultimately causing more damage to the arteries and reducing the flow of blood.

   There are three stages of coronary heart disease. First, a fatty streak appears along the lining of the vessel wall; next, the plaque builds up; and finally, the arteries harden like lead pipes.

- *Cancer:* Cancer affects one out of every four Americans. The American Cancer Society defines cancer as "a large group of diseases all characterized by uncontrolled growth and spread of abnormal cells." When normal cells mutate into abnormal cells, the body treats them like a foreign substance. One function of white blood cells is to search out and destroy these mutant cells. If, for some reason, the number of white blood cells (lymphocytes and macrophages) is too low, an abnormal cell may go undetected, and the likelihood of a tumor increases. Research suggests that the body produces about six mutant cells per day. Under normal conditions, white blood cells can do their job well. Under stressful conditions, mutant cells can go undetected and become cancerous tumors. (It should be noted that there is still much to be discovered regarding the relationship between stress and cancer.)

Prolonged stress can have a negative impact on your health. Prolonged grief, anger, or even boredom can undermine the body's physiological systems, most notably the integrity of the immune system. Current research indicates that as much as 85% of all disease and illness is stress-related. EMS professionals are potentially at a greater risk due to the exposure of repeated trauma and post-traumatic stress disorder. Remember, the body becomes the battlefield for the war-games of the mind.

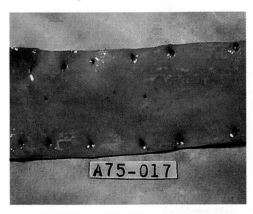

A75-017

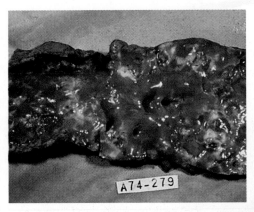

A74-279

Coronary heart disease can start as early as age 5, causing damage to the inner lining of artery walls, as shown in the second photo. Cholesterol deposits, which attempt to heal damaged tissue, actually thicken the passage, thus decreasing the diameter of the vessel for blood circulation. The greater the amount of thickness, the greater the blockage to that vessel, resulting in a heart attack.

stress | strategies

Exercise ①
Recognizing Anger

This quick exercise can help you understand how anger surfaces during a working day and how you might mismanage it. Check any of the following descriptions that apply to you when you get angry. Next, if applicable, try to identify your most common mismanaged anger style.

_____ anxious	_____ threaten others	_____ depressed
_____ buy things	_____ overeat	_____ frequent lateness
_____ start dieting	_____ never feel angry	_____ trouble sleeping
_____ tight, clenched jaw	_____ excessive sleeping	_____ bored
_____ careless driving	_____ nausea, vomiting	_____ chronic fatigue
_____ skin eruptions	_____ abuse alcohol/drugs	_____ easily irritable
_____ explode in rage	_____ sexual difficulties	_____ cold withdrawal
_____ backache	_____ headaches	_____ busywork (clean, straighten)
_____ sarcasm	_____ hostile joking	_____ sulk, whine
_____ accident-prone	_____ hit, throw things	_____ guilty and self-blaming
_____ complain and whine	_____ high blood pressure	_____ tension headaches
_____ frequent nightmares	_____ harp/nag	_____ muscle tension (e.g., shoulders, leg, fist)
_____ intellectualize	_____ name call	_____ stomach upsets (e.g., gas, cramps, colitis)
_____ cry	_____ smoke	

MISMANAGED ANGER STYLES

When I mismanage my anger, I typically express myself in the following way (check one):

_____ 1. Exploder

_____ 2. Self-punisher (guilt)

_____ 3. Underhander (revenge, sarcasm)

_____ 4. Somatizer (suppress anger feelings)

My average number of anger episodes per day is _____ .

Exercise ②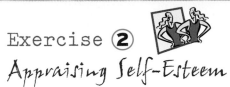

Appraising Self-Esteem

Self-esteem is often described as your sense of self-value, self-acceptance, and self-love. When your self-esteem is high, stress seems to roll off your back. When your self-esteem is low, you attract stressors like a magnet. To nurture your self-esteem, you need to address four specific areas: uniqueness, empowerment, role models, and connectedness. Take a moment to see how strong these areas are in your life right now.

I. Uniqueness. List five things about yourself that make you feel special and unique:

1.

2.

3.

4.

5.

II. Empowerment. List five areas or aspects of your life in which you feel you are in control or are self-empowered:

1.

2.

3.

4.

5.

III. Role Models. Who are your role models or mentors? Name five people who have one or more characteristics that you wish to emulate, include, or strengthen as part of your own personality and describe what that trait is.

1.

2.

3.

4.

5.

IV. Connectedness. Social support groups can be crucial to your health status. It is very important to have a sense of belonging in your life. Who (and this can include animals) do you feel you have a sense of belonging to?

1.

2.

3.

4.

5.

Exercise ③
Checking Physical Symptoms

Look over the list of stress-related symptoms and circle how often they have occurred in the past week, how severe they seemed to you, and how long they lasted. Then reflect back on the past week's workload and see whether you notice any connection.

	How Often (number of days in the past week)	How Severe (1 = mild, 5 = severe)	How Long (1 = 1 hour, 5 = all day)
1. Tension headache	0 1 2 3 4 5 6 7	1 2 3 4 5	1 2 3 4 5
2. Migraine headache	0 1 2 3 4 5 6 7	1 2 3 4 5	1 2 3 4 5
3. Muscle tension (neck and/or shoulders)	0 1 2 3 4 5 6 7	1 2 3 4 5	1 2 3 4 5
4. Muscle tension (lower back)	0 1 2 3 4 5 6 7	1 2 3 4 5	1 2 3 4 5
5. Joint pain	0 1 2 3 4 5 6 7	1 2 3 4 5	1 2 3 4 5
6. Cold	0 1 2 3 4 5 6 7	1 2 3 4 5	1 2 3 4 5
7. Flu	0 1 2 3 4 5 6 7	1 2 3 4 5	1 2 3 4 5
8. Stomachache	0 1 2 3 4 5 6 7	1 2 3 4 5	1 2 3 4 5
9. Stomach/abdominal bloating/distention/gas	0 1 2 3 4 5 6 7	1 2 3 4 5	1 2 3 4 5
10. Diarrhea	0 1 2 3 4 5 6 7	1 2 3 4 5	1 2 3 4 5
11. Constipation	0 1 2 3 4 5 6 7	1 2 3 4 5	1 2 3 4 5
12. Ulcer flare-up	0 1 2 3 4 5 6 7	1 2 3 4 5	1 2 3 4 5
13. Asthma attack	0 1 2 3 4 5 6 7	1 2 3 4 5	1 2 3 4 5
14. Allergies	0 1 2 3 4 5 6 7	1 2 3 4 5	1 2 3 4 5
15. Canker/cold sores	0 1 2 3 4 5 6 7	1 2 3 4 5	1 2 3 4 5
16. Dizzy spells	0 1 2 3 4 5 6 7	1 2 3 4 5	1 2 3 4 5
17. Heart palpitations (racing heart)	0 1 2 3 4 5 6 7	1 2 3 4 5	1 2 3 4 5

Exercise ③
Checking Physical Symptoms—continued

	How Often (number of days in the past week)	How Severe (1 = mild, 5 = severe)	How Long (1 = 1 hour, 5 = all day)
18. TMJ	0 1 2 3 4 5 6 7	1 2 3 4 5	1 2 3 4 5
19. Insomnia	0 1 2 3 4 5 6 7	1 2 3 4 5	1 2 3 4 5
20. Nightmares	0 1 2 3 4 5 6 7	1 2 3 4 5	1 2 3 4 5
21. Fatigue	0 1 2 3 4 5 6 7	1 2 3 4 5	1 2 3 4 5
22. Hemorrhoids	0 1 2 3 4 5 6 7	1 2 3 4 5	1 2 3 4 5
23. Pimples/acne	0 1 2 3 4 5 6 7	1 2 3 4 5	1 2 3 4 5
24. Cramps	0 1 2 3 4 5 6 7	1 2 3 4 5	1 2 3 4 5
25. Frequent accidents	0 1 2 3 4 5 6 7	1 2 3 4 5	1 2 3 4 5
26. Other (please specify):	0 1 2 3 4 5 6 7	1 2 3 4 5	1 2 3 4 5

Score: Take a look at the entire list. Do you observe any patterns or relationships between your stress levels and your physical health? A value over 30 points (in all 3 areas combined) could indicate a stress-related health problem. If it seems to you that these symptoms are related to undue stress, they probably are. You should seek medical treatment when necessary, and you may want to consider the regular use of relaxation techniques to help lessen the intensity, frequency, and duration of these episodes.

Score _____		
	0 - 10 points :	low stress reaction
	11 - 20 points :	moderate stress reaction
	21 - 30 points :	moderately high stress reaction
	Over 30 points :	high stress reaction*

* It might be a good idea to seek some counseling about this.

Chapter 3 Effective Coping Skills

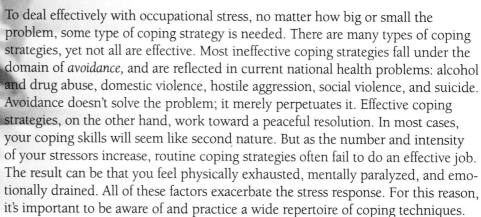

Anyone who knows Jim will tell you he has a warped (some say sick) sense of humor, but Jim will tell you it's the one thing that gets him through a grim day.

Jim's not alone; many EMTs share his dark sense of comic relief. When Scott isn't fighting fires, he's often in his workshop tying flies or off on a fly fishing trip. Carol, a dispatcher, belongs to a roadrunner's club; she runs for the camaraderie more than the exercise. Josh, a state director, feels the same about his mountain biking group. Humor, hobbies, and support groups are just a few of the ways that people use to cope with the pressures of life, and particularly to balance the stress from work. Successful coping techniques help you stay grounded and centered during a hectic day.

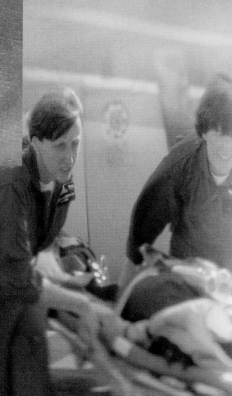

How many psychologists does it take to change a light bulb? One! But the light bulb has really got to want to change.

Anonymous

To deal effectively with occupational stress, no matter how big or small the problem, some type of coping strategy is needed. There are many types of coping strategies, yet not all are effective. Most ineffective coping strategies fall under the domain of *avoidance,* and are reflected in current national health problems: alcohol and drug abuse, domestic violence, hostile aggression, social violence, and suicide. Avoidance doesn't solve the problem; it merely perpetuates it. Effective coping strategies, on the other hand, work toward a peaceful resolution. In most cases, your coping skills will seem like second nature. But as the number and intensity of your stressors increase, routine coping strategies often fail to do an effective job. The result can be that you feel physically exhausted, mentally paralyzed, and emotionally drained. All of these factors exacerbate the stress response. For this reason, it's important to be aware of and practice a wide repertoire of coping techniques.

Effective coping is defined as "the mental process of managing demands that are appraised as a challenge to your resources." Coping requires both internal and external resources. Creativity, patience, optimism, intuition, a sense of humor, will power, and compassion are examples of internal resources. External resources include time, money, and social support.

Coping strategies that successfully deal with stress involve four basic components:

1. *Increased awareness of the problem:* A clear, objective focus and full perspective on the situation at hand.
2. *Information processing:* A shift in your perception to deactivate the threat. Information processing also includes gathering and assessing all resources available in order to resolve the problem.
3. *Changing behaviors:* Consciously chosen actions that, combined with a positive attitude, can dissolve, minimize, or eradicate the stressor.
4. *Peaceful resolution:* A feeling that the situation has successfully been brought to closure.

The goal of effective coping skills is to maintain a sense of mental and emotional equilibrium under the constraints of professional challenges and obligations, as well as personal pressures—in other words, not merely to survive from one day to the next, but to thrive in the face of adversity, to be the victor, not the victim. Research suggests that there is no one-size-fits-all approach to coping with stress. The best strategy is to be aware of several different coping methods and to cultivate these skills regularly so that they are available immediately when needed.

Is there a relationship between the use of effective coping strategies and personality at the worksite? Some researchers think so. People who have stress-prone personalities, such as the Type A (people who are aggressive with hostile anger), Codependent (approval-seeking perfectionists), and Helpless-Hopeless (people with rock bottom self-esteem) behaviors, are more likely to choose and employ negative coping styles by avoiding problems and claiming victimization. People who exhibit stress-resistant personality traits, such as the Hardy Personality (people with resilient personalities based upon a high level of commitment, control, and challenge) and the Sensation Seeker (people who live for the moment, but only take calculated risks), are more likely to see challenges rather than threats, take calculated risks, diplomatically confront rather than avoid problems, and quickly resolve their stressors. It goes without saying that EMS professionals tend to have personalities that lend themselves to repeated challenges. However, the hardiest personality stays that way by practicing the skills of effective coping techniques.

A single coping technique is rarely used alone. Rather, several skills are used *collectively* to build a stronger defense against stress. Some coping strategies, such as reframing, information seeking, creative problem solving, journal writing, and humor therapy, help you understand and deal with your problems. Other coping skills emphasize a thinking strategy combined with a conscious change in behavior. These include time management, assertiveness skills, communication skills, social engineering, and hobbies. Your skill in using coping techniques will improve with practice. It is important to remember that no one coping technique will work as a defense against all types of stress, so you should have many coping skills from which to choose to make your life less stressful. This chapter is divided into two parts: personal coping skills (refining your cognitive perceptions) and interpersonal coping skills (refining your interpersonal skills).

> **Effective Coping Strategies =**
>
> **Increased Awareness**
> +
> **Information Processing**
> +
> **Modified Behavior**
> +
> **Peaceful Resolution**

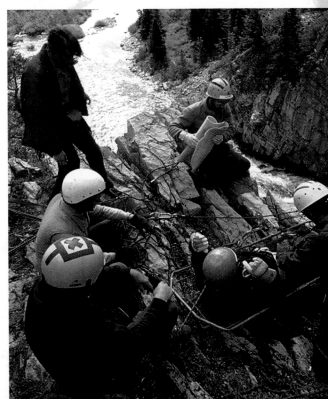

Personal coping skills such as reframing and creative problem solving can also help you in your professional life.

Personal Coping Skills

Reframing Stressful Thoughts

Excessive overtime hours. A drunk belligerent perpetrator. Numerous reports to file. A call in the middle of your anniversary dinner. A long distant transport. Stressors come in all shapes and sizes. It is not the circumstance or environment that is stressful, but rather the *perception* or interpretation of the situation. If the perception is negative, it can become both a mental and physical liability. Whatever the event, perceptions can magnify and distort it entirely out of proportion and turn everyday problems into catastrophic monsters. By learning to reframe your perceptions, you can avoid the pitfalls of toxic thoughts.

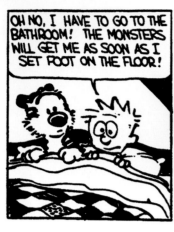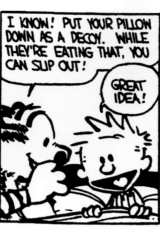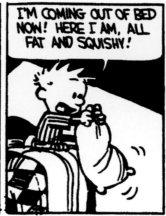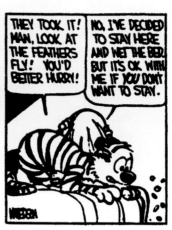

Whether stress is imaginary or real, it can cause a stress response in the body.

Toxic Thoughts

Self-talk is a never-ending conversation running through your head. Most self-talk consists of negative thoughts, criticisms, and put-downs, or what are often referred to as *toxic thoughts*. Toxic thoughts are directly related to low self-esteem.

Toxic thoughts perpetuate the cycle of low self-esteem by ignoring or destroying feelings of self-worth and self-acceptance. Negative thoughts are actually a response learned in childhood that carries into adult life. Studies show that a pessimistic attitude that generates toxic thoughts also makes people more prone to disease and illness. On the other hand, an optimistic attitude promotes a great sense of well-being. In short, toxic thoughts can have a toxic effect on the body and put your health at risk. For example, studies on the longevity of cancer patients with breast cancer show that patients with a "fighting spirit" are more likely to live longer than those who appear to "give in" and "give up" (every documented case of a miracle cure has been accompanied by a positive change in attitude). Furthermore, negative thoughts influence negative actions in what is called the *"self-fulfilling prophecy."* In order for you to raise your self-esteem, you need to change, or reframe, these toxic thoughts. Quite often, stubbornness and the comfort of your own opinions become obstacles to changing toxic thoughts. Think of how you can change the dialogue in your mind so that you produce fewer toxic thoughts while you are at work in the station or the field.

Adopt a Positive Attitude

Reframing is a coping technique that favorably changes a stressful attitude to a less threatening perception—in other words, from a negative, self-defeating attitude to a positive attitude. In every moment, you choose your attitude toward life and its challenges. The purpose of reframing is to widen your perspective and focus on the positive aspects of challenging situations. The ability to see more than what is directly in front of you is not merely a poetic expression. It has been proven that, like tunnel vision, your field of vision actually narrows under stress. When your imagination is limited, so too are your possibilities for dealing with the situation.

Reframing should not be confused with rationalization. Rationalization is an ego defense mechanism that makes excuses, blames others, and shifts the responsibility away from yourself toward someone or something else. Reframing allows you to find and adopt a positive mind frame to deal with any unpleasant situation involving your work. Reframing does not deny you the ability to mourn, grieve, or experience negative thoughts that result from stress. Nor is reframing an overly optimistic, "Pollyanna" attitude. It does, however, help you break the cycle of negative thinking that can block the path to resolution. Tools to initiate the reframing

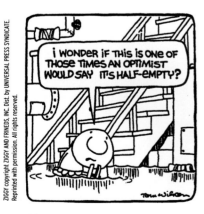

It is normal to have negative thoughts, but too many too often can result in a pessimistic outlook, which only creates more stress.

For Your Information

Toxic Thoughts

Toxic thoughts can appear in the following ways:

1. **Pessimism:** Casting a negative perspective on almost every situation.

2. **Catastrophizing:** Imagining the worst of a situation, always seeing everything as awful.

3. **Blaming:** Shifting the responsibility of circumstances to someone other than yourself.

4. **Perfectionism:** Imposing above-human standards on yourself or others, expecting everything you or they do to be perfect.

5. **Polarized thinking:** Seeing everything as extremes (either good or bad, black or white, etc.) with no middle ground.

6. **Should-ing:** Reprimanding yourself for things you "should" have done.

7. **Victimization:** Feeling as though you have been singled out and taken advantage of by other people, events, or circumstances.

---

process and dismantle the obstacles include the use of humor, positive affirmations, and creativity. One major element of the reframing process that is designed to bolster self-esteem is the use of positive affirmations: "I am confident" or "I am doing the best I can." Confidence building through positive self-talk can counterbalance the voice of the "inner critic," the voice in your head that constantly tells you that you're just not good enough.

> When you have absolutely no control over the outcome, you must learn to accept the situation as it is and move on.

Acceptance: An Alternative Mind Frame

Often you encounter situations over which you have no control: a malfunctioning piece of equipment during a rescue, a traffic jam, or poor weather conditions. The reality of the situation is not pleasant. But you can waste a lot of personal energy trying to change things over which you have no control. The weather and the behavior of others are just two examples. When you have absolutely no control over the outcome, you must learn to accept the situation as it is and move on. Moving on can mean exploring and trying other options, or simply putting your hands at rest, knowing that there is nothing more that you can do. There is a fine balance between control and acceptance, and acceptance should not be confused with apathy or surrender. Acceptance is perhaps the hardest frame of mind to adopt. It does not happen overnight; it is an attitude that might take days, weeks, or even months to adopt, depending on the nature of the stressor. But in some cases, acceptance is the only choice. A rescue that results in death is not a failed rescue. In the larger picture, there is an agenda in which we participate but do not control. These words by Reinhold Neibuhr are good to remember: "Grant me the serenity to accept the things I cannot change, the courage to change the things I can, and the wisdom to know the difference."

Steps to Initiate Reframing

You can use reframing as a coping technique. Think of a situation at work and try this four-step approach:

1. *Increase your awareness:* Identify your stressor by asking yourself what is bothering you. (Exercise 1 at the end of the chapter helps you identify your stressors.) Try writing down what is on your mind, including all your fears, frustrations, and/or worries.

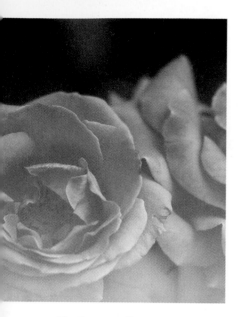

Situations can offer both positive and negative experiences, like a rose that has both petals and thorns. Where do you choose to place your attention?

2. *Reframe your perception:* Create a positive reference toward this one circumstance by finding something positive about the situation.

3. *Adopt this new attitude:* Try to focus on the positive and minimize the negative aspects of the problem. If you cannot find anything positive, what valuable aspect can you learn from the experience?

4. *Evaluate:* Make an assessment of your new attitude and ask yourself "Did this help?" If it turns out that this was a complete failure, then go back to the cause of the problem and find something else about the situation that is positive. Even the worst situations offer valuable lessons. Take the time to learn these lessons.

Here are some additional tips on reframing:

1. *Disarm the negative critic:* Stop the negative conversation in your head. When you become aware of your negative self-talk, say to yourself, "Stop this thought," and then focus your attention on one of your positive attributes.

2. *Take responsibility for your own thoughts:* If you find yourself blaming others for events that make you feel hurt, ask yourself how you can turn this blame into personal responsibility for your own thoughts and feelings without feeling guilty.

3. *Fine tune your expectations:* Sometimes, you walk into a situation with a preconceived attitude or expectation. When your expectations are not met to your satisfaction, negative feelings are generated. Fine-tuning your expectations doesn't mean abandoning your ideals. Rather, it means giving your perceptions a reality check, questioning their validity, and matching them to the situation.

4. *Give yourself positive affirmations:* Positive affirmations provide you with good thoughts to enhance your self-confidence and self-esteem. Use a phrase that when repeated to yourself, boosts your self-esteem, such as "I am a caring person" or "I can do it."

5. *Accentuate the positive:* There is a difference between positive thinking and focusing on the positive. Positive thinking is an expression of hope for future events. It is often characterized by goal setting, wishful thinking, and dreaming. Positive thinking can be healthy, but it can also be a form of denial if done in excess. Focusing on the positive is reframing the current situation. It is an appreciation of the present moment. Acknowledge the negative and learn from it, but don't dwell on it. Focus on the positive aspects and build on them. As with a rose that has both petals and thorns, you can choose where to focus your attention. As a personal example, find five positive aspects of the first problem you listed in Exercise 1.

Ultimately, you are responsible for the creation of your own thoughts. Shifting our thoughts from a negative stance to a positive attitude is necessary to break the cycle of perceptions that promote stressful threats.

Comic Relief: Humor Therapy

www.StressLessEMS.com

People who frequently encounter death and dying often use humor to soften the emotional blow of trauma and tragedy. This brand of humor, commonly known as "gallows humor" or "black humor," is best defined as humor that makes fun of a disastrous or terrifying situation. The

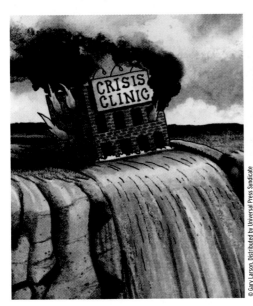

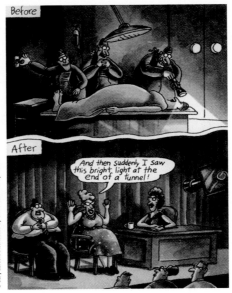

Black humor is a common way to cope with repeated exposure to death and dying.

television show *M*A*S*H* and movies such as *Harold and Maude, Eating Raoul,* and *Heathers* used black humor. While these jokes might seem bizarre, rude, shocking, or in poor taste to some people, those who work on the front lines of death and dying know that this humor style serves to calm nerves in very tense situations. A quick wit, a sense of irony, and puns are other humorous approaches that can be used on duty and during the decompression period afterward.

The healing power of humor as a viable coping technique dates back to antiquity. Ever since Norman Cousins laughed himself back to health from a life-threatening disease in 1964, the use of humor or comic relief has gained wide recognition as a way of effectively coping with stress. On average, Americans laugh 15 times per day, yet under chronic stress, your laughter level can drop to zero. The use of humor can help to relieve the tension of anger when you can take a moment to laugh at your misfortunes and mistakes. Humor can be used to dilute your sense of fear as well, which is why gallows humor is so effective. Humor therapists agree that humor, like stress, is a perception. When you attempt to look at the humorous side of life, you tend to inoculate yourself against the hazards of stressful perceptions.

It is important to remember that a humorous approach should not be self-deprecating or lower your own self-esteem; nor should humor, particularly sarcasm, be used to direct anger at others. Think of some ways in which you can use elements of humor to lift your spirits at work and help you reach your quota of 15 humorous moments a day (for example, listening to a humorous radio program on your way to work, sharing funny stories, or collecting cartoon panels for the bulletin board).

Hobbies

Every now and then, you need to take a break from life's pressures. Healthy diversions offer a temporary escape from the sensory overload that can perpetuate or produce the stress response. Taking your mind off a problem by diverting your attention to an unrelated subject can actually focus your mind and enable it to deal better with the issue later. Hobbies or active escapes contribute to your identity, character, and self-esteem. Most hobbies, whether photography, rock climbing, scuba diving, or fly tying, include some degree of creativity as well as the ability to make order out of chaos on a small, manageable scale. This can

Hobbies are an ideal temporary escape from everyday stress.

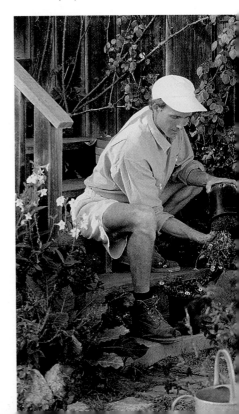

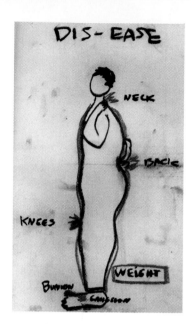

DIS-EASE

NECK

BACK

KNEES

WEIGHT

Art therapy can help you release harmful thoughts, and bring the body back toward homeostasis.

give you a sense of control over life, which in turn augments self-esteem. High self-esteem transfers from outside interests to areas of your life in which these factors contribute to personal success. Moreover, the ability to bring order to a small-scale operation, such as haute cuisine cooking or bonsai gardening, also has a carryover effect in dealing with larger work-related problems. Right now, make a list of three hobbies you are engaged in. (Watching television is not a hobby!) If you don't have any hobbies, what is one area of interest you would like to get involved in?

Journal Writing and Art Therapy

StressLess EMS

www.StressLessEMS.com

Keeping thoughts and feelings caused by repeated exposure to traumatic events inside can have some devastating effects. By cleansing your mind of these thoughts and feelings through writing or art, you lay a foundation for a better sense of harmony among mind, body, and spirit.

Studies by James Pennebaker at Southern Methodist University show that by getting thoughts, feelings, and images onto paper, the unconscious mind is less troubled and more calm; this in turn enhances the immune system. Although your schedule might not allow you to sit down every day after work and compose a four- to five-page essay about your work experiences, this might not be a bad option if you have problems sleeping, wake from a dream in the middle of the night, or just feel fidgety or down in the dumps. Expressing yourself through words or pictures can be very cathartic (the emotional equivalent of letting down a heavy load). You don't have to be Ernest Hemingway to take pen to paper; nor do you have to be Da Vinci to be an artist. The benefit in writing or drawing is not in the outcome, but in the process of letting go. The result is a greater sense of calm because the toxic thoughts and feelings that were once captive in your mind are free. Exercise 2 is a sample journal theme, and Exercise 3 is a sample art therapy theme. If these are coping techniques that you think might help you, give them a try.

Creative Problem Solving

It would be nice if every rescue or emergency response followed textbook protocol, but the truth is that things can and will go wrong. Machine failures, equipment breakdowns, and miscalculations are a reality of EMS. The life and care of your patient may hinge on your creative insights, spontaneous ingenuity, quick mind, and excellent creative skills. The Apollo 13 mission was a case of distant emergency response, when NASA engineers on earth had to devise a rescue plan (which turned out to be composed of plastic bags, pipes, and duct tape). While your rescues might not be as dramatic as this one, the concepts of creative problem solving are the same. Whether you have to disarm a patient who has a handgun or set a broken femur with no splints, you need to keep your creative muscles in good shape for everyday preparedness.

Creativity, the mother of invention and the father of play, is talent that resides within everyone. Creativity is not a gift; it is a human birthright. But creativity must be regularly exercised to be effective or it will shrink with disuse, just like any other muscle. Stress is often

Tense situations often foster the need for quick thinking. The team in the Mission Operations Control Room of the Apollo 13 mission showed creativity in helping the astronauts get back safely.

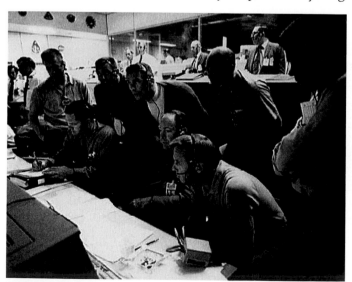

defined as "any change in your environment," and creativity has the ability to make change palatable, perhaps even enjoyable. But creativity takes the right attitude and a workable strategy. Creativity can be one of your most important stress management tools at work or home. Here's a look at the basics of creativity.

The Creative Process
In simple terms, the creative process has two parts: *primary creativity* (or right brain function) and *secondary creativity* (left brain function). Primary creativity is the idea originator. It is the "playground of the mind" where ideas are generated and hatched. Secondary creativity creates the strategic plan to ripen those ideas. Secondary creativity is the mind's workshop: a place to saw, chisel, glue, hammer, and polish ideas for functional use.

In his book *A Kick in the Seat of the Pants,* creativity consultant Roger von Oech elaborates even further by describing the creative process as a combination of four phases: the *Explorer,* the *Artist,* the *Judge,* and the *Warrior.* The Explorer and Artist serve in the capacity of primary creativity, and the Judge and the Warrior serve in the roles of secondary creativity. In the creative process, each player should do its job without interference from the other three. The goal of creative processing is to sharpen the skills of all four team players, so that one or two aspects don't overpower the others or stifle the entire creative process.

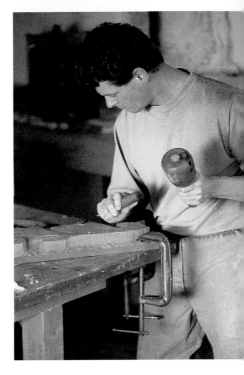

Many hobbies offer ways to explore creative outlets.

1. *The Explorer:* The Explorer searches for raw materials to create ideas. The most important equipment the Explorer needs is an open mind: a container in which to put the raw materials. Negative thoughts close a mind water-tight. An open mind employs several attitudes, such as curiosity, optimism, and enthusiasm, as fertilizers for ideas. To get new ideas, the Explorer must explore territories outside the normal bounds and comfort zone of everyday life. For example, subscribing to a magazine outside your professional field, visiting an art museum, or roaming the aisles of a hardware store can all sow the seeds of creativity.

2. *The Artist:* In the Artist phase, the raw materials (ideas) are cultivated, manipulated, and sometimes incubated until they are molded into functional use. If the Explorer asks "Where?," then the Artist asks "How and what?" In the role of the artist, you play with ideas and begin to turn them into real possibilities.

3. *The Judge:* The Judge casts a thumbs up or down decision for each idea, and the good ideas are kept to become reality. The role of the Judge is crucial, for the Judge can destroy good ideas as easily as it can make good ideas really happen. Critical thoughts and overanalysis used at the wrong time can dominate and destroy the other stages, resulting in a waste of both time and resources. In the North American culture, the Judge (a left brain skill) is often the strongest player in the creative team.

4. *The Warrior:* The Warrior, in tandem with the Judge, takes the creative idea "to the streets." Like a quarterback, the Warrior creates an action plan, a winning game plan. There is a saying on Wall Street that goes like this: "To know and not to do is not to know." Warrior skills require good organization and administration abilities.

The Creative Process

The Problem

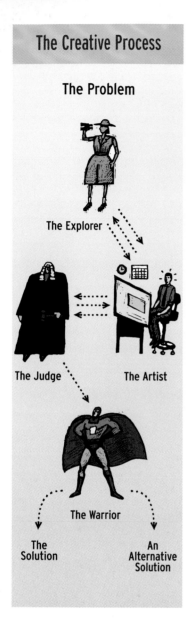

The Explorer

The Judge   The Artist

The Warrior

The   An
Solution   Alternative
                 Solution

Creativity is a nonlinear process.

Creative Problem Solving in Acute Stress Situations

Critical emergency care does not always allow the luxury of extended time to make creative problem-solving decisions. You might have only seconds to reach a decision. The same template of creative roles can be used, but the process looks more like intuition. The ability to make fast creative decisions is a process that combines clear thinking, wisdom based on any and all past experiences, and sudden insight from the depths of the unconscious mind. Aspects of this creative process can be cultivated during slow times by playing the game "What if?" Create a scenario that taxes your creative skills and play with alternatives. For example, what if the battery pack on the defibrillator is dead? What if the patient who needs transport weighs 500 pounds?

Roadblocks to Creativity

There are many reasons why the creative process gets ignored. Obstacles to creativity begin with negative attitudes perpetuating the myth that only a chosen few are truly gifted. This attitude eventually promotes a sense of creative laziness. Some popular attitudes that inhibit the creative process, as noted by von Oech, include the following:

1. *I'm not creative:* Creativity isn't a perception. It is a process. Everyone is creative; it just takes some effort. What separates people like Picasso, Madonna, and Walt Disney from those who say they are not creative? The main difference is the belief these people have in themselves that they *are* creative. See yourself as an untapped wellspring of creativity and you can begin to use your creativity.

2. *There is only one right answer:* The typical attitude in many cultures is that there is only one right answer to every problem. Once the apparent answer is found, everyone stops looking. In the germination phase of the creative process there are many real possibilities. If you search for one right answer, you will surely stop once you think you have found it. For solving work-related problems, nothing could be more dangerous.

3. *Don't be foolish:* To avoid seeming foolish in front of others, you may keep your guard up. Guarded behavior promotes conformity, which in turn breeds staleness. In the creative process, this mentality can lead to a concept called "group think," in which everyone conforms and goes along with

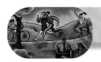

road to relaxation

Creativity Motivational Quotes

"Nothing is more dangerous than an idea when it is the only one you have."
Emile Chartier

"Every act of creation is first an act of destruction."
Picasso

"The best way to get a good idea is to get a lot of ideas."
Linus Pauling

"Afflict the Comfortable, Comfort the Afflicted."
Carl Ally

"If your only tool is a hammer, you'll see every problem as a nail."
Abraham Maslow

"A ship in port is safe, but that's not what ships are built for."
Grace Hopper

"If you do not ask 'why this?' often enough, somebody will ask, 'why you?'"
Tom Hirshfield

"Slaying sacred cows makes great steaks!"
Dick Nicolosi

the crowd. Group think is considered dangerous because it stifles creativity. Sometimes, you need to give yourself permission to be foolish. A giddy outlook gives you a new perspective on a situation. Playing the fool can assist the Judge in determining the worthiness of ideas. Being foolish can also mean using your sense of humor, which in itself is a great coping technique.

4. *Avoid mistakes:* There are times when making a mistake is not a good idea. It might cost you your job, marriage, or life. Then again, there are times when making a mistake might result in the most appropriate course of action. Mistakes can teach us how *not to do* something. Early in the creative process, mistakes are necessary. Each mistake clears a path to a more viable answer. The fear of failure can immobilize the creative process. Don't let it!

From Creativity to Creative Problem Solving

As a coping technique, creativity is perhaps *the* most valuable weapon to use in your personal battle against stress. Not only does creativity boost your self-esteem, but the more options you have for solving a problem, the better are your chances of reducing stress. At first glance, creative problem solving might appear to be a linear process for getting from point A to point B. In reality, the problem-solving process is more roundabout.

Steps to Initiate Creative Problem Solving

You can use a five-point strategy to initiate the creative process to untangle personal and professional problems:

1. *Describe the problem:* Before you can attack a problem successfully, you have to understand it. State the problem objectively. Define it. Next, analyze the problem. Dissect it. Look at its components. What are its strengths and weaknesses? What is the face value and what is the bottom line?

2. *Generate ideas:* Generating ideas is fun and challenging. You can get ideas from any available resource, both internal and external: books, people, movies, museums, memory—you name it! This is where the Explorer role comes in. The more ideas you have, the better your chances are to solve the problem effectively. When searching for ideas, leave the mind's censorship role behind. Don't judge and discard immediately.

road to relaxation

Creativity Motivational Quotes—continued.

"No one ever achieved greatness by playing it safe."
Harry Gray

"To know and not to do, is not to know."
Wall Street Slogan

"The only person who likes change is a wet baby."
Roy Blitzer

"If you are not failing every now and again, it is a sign that you're not trying anything very innovative."
Woody Allen

"The way to success is to double your rate of failure."
Thomas J. Watson (IBM founder)

"Discovery consists of looking at the same thing as everyone else and thinking something different."
Albert Györgyi

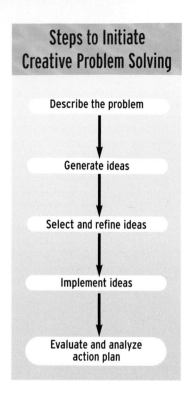

Steps to Initiate Creative Problem Solving

Describe the problem

↓

Generate ideas

↓

Select and refine ideas

↓

Implement ideas

↓

Evaluate and analyze action plan

3. *Select and refine your ideas:* Not all ideas will be good or usable. Once your ideas are laid out, one or two will jump out at you as the most likely to succeed. Rank the order (the Judge) of these ideas according to their degree of feasibility (plan A, plan B, plan C, etc.). Once you have made your selection, begin to manipulate the idea to suit the problem. This might mean streamlining the idea or making some alterations to address your direct needs.

4. *Implement the idea(s):* Implementation involves both a strategy and an element of risk. Ask yourself, "How can this idea be put into effect to resolve the problem?" Implementation means making a game plan to try the idea out, to see whether it floats or sinks. In addition to bravery (risk taking), implementation requires faith; an idea without faith is like a car without wheels.

5. *Evaluate and analyze the action:* A good inventor watches to see how well his or her invention works. When the series of tests is through, either a bottle of champagne is opened or there's a return trip to the drawing board. The final lesson a problem has to offer is whether it was resolved and *how well* it was resolved.

You have the skills to be creative. The question is whether or not you choose to use them. In an effort to explain the importance of creativity, psychologist Abraham Maslow once said, "People who are only good with hammers see every problem as a nail." He was convinced that creativity is the necessary skill to deal with the stress of change. As a coping technique, creativity is the only choice if you want to deal effectively with stress. Creative problem-solving skills are life skills: skills that will help you not only survive, but thrive in the chaos of change. These skills, once refined, can and should be used repeatedly in confronting and resolving stress.

www.StressLessEMS.com

Dream Therapy

Dreams might seem like an insignificant part of your life, but dreams may convey ideas that can help you solve problems in the awake state. Perhaps of greatest importance to EMS professionals are the dreams that surface as a result of dangerous work situations. Also important are recurring dreams that convey a situation begging to be resolved. Dream therapy—the process of remembering, exploring and interpreting your dreams—is one way to gain "psychic equilibrium," the mental and emotional balance between the conscious and unconscious minds. In dream therapy, you try to recall dreams of the previous night and write down whatever remnants or dream fragments you can recall. You then process the dream information by looking at both the literal and the symbolic messages. The language of dreams is a foreign language until we become more fluent in the symbols of the images. Recurring dreams may be an unconscious acknowledgement of some unresolved issue. One technique you can use is *active imagination.* When you awake, write down the recurring dream in as much detail as possible, then write an ending to the dream, again with as much detail as possible. By doing this, you can begin to work resolving the issue both consciously and unconsciously. Exercise 5 gives you a chance to explore the resolutions of recurring dreams.

Time Management

Everyone has time management issues, from the corporate executive who works with project deadlines to the secretary who is overwhelmed with tasks assigned by five supervisors. You, as an EMS professional, have very different scenarios with regard to time management. How can you balance the time constraints between your professional career and your personal life? Irregular shifts, overtime requests, and other issues can cause your personal life to suffer, perhaps even beginning a downward spiral toward marital problems, divorce, or other personal disasters. As an EMS professional, you make yourself available to serve others, but your home life could probably use some compassionate assistance as well.

Good time management skills in the field, at the station, or at home involve two aspects. First, be aware of time wasters, activities or behaviors that rob you of valuable time. Second, learn organizational skills that allow you to prioritize, schedule, and execute personal responsibilities to your personal satisfaction. Good time management skills incorporate good boundaries and high self-esteem, recognizing that you deserve a balance between your personal and professional life. This section will first examine time wasters, or "time robbers," and then offer tips on how to prioritize, schedule, and execute your personal responsibilities to the highest level of personal satisfaction.

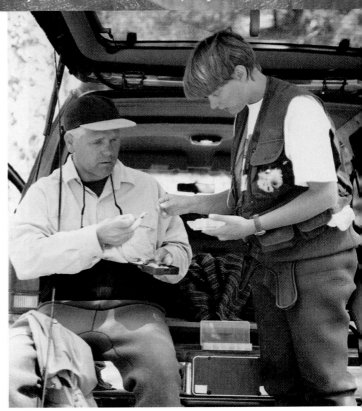

Good time management includes scheduling time for your personal life.

Time Wasters/Time Robbers

Four common behaviors are noted as "time robbers" because they steal valuable time, rather than promoting effective time usage. As you read, determine whether any apply to you.

- *Poor personal boundaries:* Some people have a hard time saying no to friends and co-workers (a common trait among professional caregivers). This leaves no time for yourself, your spouse, or family members. You may feel as though others are taking advantage of you.

- *Workaholism:* Workaholics commonly spend more time, but not necessarily productive time, on the job, usually to compensate for low self-esteem. A person might spend more hours on the job to feel more important.

- *Procrastination:* Procrastination is a diversion tactic to avoid responsibilities. Four factors are associated with procrastination: laziness, apathy, the fear of failure, and the need for instant gratification. Procrastinators end up rushing to do a job that they really had plenty of time to do. In most cases, work takes priority over home responsibilities, and family members or family obligations suffer.

- *Perfectionism:* The perfectionist shows near-obsessive, even compulsive, behavior by attempting to complete every task and responsibility to perfection. While safety issues certainly require attentiveness to several factors, the perfectionist goes beyond the extra mile to clean up or attend to the very last detail.

Time Management Techniques

One of the best definitions of time management is, "The ability to prioritize, schedule, and execute personal responsibilities to personal satisfaction." If your time seems hard to manage, ask yourself which of these areas (prioritization, scheduling, or execution) needs your attention. The current trend in time management involves focus, as in Steven Covey's idea of "first things first, and deletion, removing any and all things that crowd one's lifestyle and impede getting things done (e.g., abundant television viewing)."

Listening and Responding Skills

❶ Assume the role of a listener.

❷ Maintain eye contact.

❸ Avoid word prejudice.

❹ Use minimal encouragers.

❺ Paraphrase the content of what was said to ensure clarification.

❻ Ask questions to clarify statements.

❼ Use empathy to reflect and share the individual's feelings.

❽ Provide personal feedback.

❾ Summarize the content of what was said.

3. *Avoid word prejudice:* Some words can elicit obvious emotional responses in which the listener begins to show signs of indifference or surprise. Words that refer to political allegiances or religious beliefs can press buttons and set the emotional wheels spinning. Raised eyebrows, frowns, and side glances are overt signs of word prejudice. Please be careful how you use these types of words.

4. *Use minimal encouragers:* Minimal encouragers indicate that you are on the same wavelength as the speaker. They include the use of short word phrases such as "oh?" or "uh-huh?" or repeating key words to encourage the person to give you more detailed information about the subject. Remember, these encouragers should be used genuinely, not mechanically.

5. *Paraphrase the content of what was said to ensure clarification:* Paraphrasing is a more elaborate style of minimal encouragement. In addition to repeating key words, paraphrasing includes adding your observations to show that you understand the content of message.

6. *Ask questions to clarify statements:* When you can't understand facts, concepts, or feelings being expressed, ask questions. You want to understand what the other person is saying. Don't be afraid to ask people to explain what they mean. But beware: Questions can sometimes put the speaker on the defensive. Use questions to clarify your understanding, not to confuse the speaker.

7. *Use empathy to reflect and share the individual's feelings:* Empathy is thought to be an important attending skill. Empathy refers to the selective attention given to the individual's feelings as well as his or her thoughts. Empathy does not imply that you adopt these feelings as your own. Rather, empathy lets you recognize the speaker's feelings.

8. *Provide personal feedback:* Responding to comments often requires feedback from the listener. Before you offer your opinion, ask whether feedback is desired. If your viewpoint is invited, offer your comments and criticism in a constructive way, balancing positive aspects with negative perceptions. Provide details and insights aimed at improving the situation.

9. *Summarize the content of what was said:* Summarizing is similar to paraphrasing but requires more concentration and synthesis of the other person's thoughts and feelings to fully comprehend what was said. This is really important in describing details of a job.

Steps to Enhance Communication Skills

These additional suggestions can help strengthen your communication skills and promote conflict resolution:

1. *Speak with precision and directness:* Be as direct as possible in expressing your thoughts and perceptions. Select words that accurately express how you feel. Clearly state the intention of your message.

2. *Enhance your vocabulary:* A small vocabulary can limit your ability to express yourself. If you can choose from a wide selection of words (especially adjectives and adverbs), you will have greater flexibility in expressing yourself clearly.

3. *Use language that is appropriate for your listening audience:* The way you speak with a service director might differ considerably from the way you talk with a squad member. Assess what words, expressions, and gestures are most conducive to explaining what you really want to say.

4. *Attack issues, not people:* When trying to resolve conflicts, focus on the problems and not the people. Avoid character assassination. Attacking people tends to raise other concerns that cloud the issue. It can be harder, if not impossible, to resolve issues when people are on the defensive. When you are wrong, apologize.

5. *Avoid putting others on the defensive:* When you initiate self-disclosure or a dialogue to resolve conflicts, begin your statements with the words, "I perceive the problem this way...." By placing the responsibility of understanding on yourself, rather than blaming others, you minimize the chance of putting others on the defensive and prolonging the conflict.

6. *Avoid indirect communication (asking someone else to pass on your thoughts or intentions to a third party):* The most effective communication is direct contact. Involving a third party (e.g., "Ask my partner to switch shifts with me") not only increases the chances for miscommunication of the intended message, it also sends nonverbal messages.

7. *Avoid information overload:* Pace your conversation to allow people ample time to understand the information that you are conveying. Avoid overloading them with too much information at once.

8. *Double-check your assumptions:* Many episodes of miscommunication result from incorrect assumptions. Even if you are sure about information or ideas from another person, it is always best to validate your perceptions before you act on them. This saves both emotional energy and, in the long run, time.

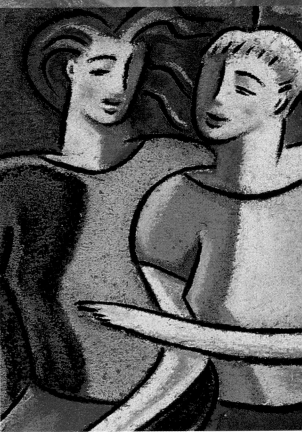

Make it a habit to practice good communication skills.

9. *Resolve issues when they arise:* If you feel that a misunderstanding exists, you're probably right. Try to deal with issues as they surface, by talking them out with those involved. Be assertive. Indicate that there is a problem, if you believe there is one. Avoiding issues or letting them fester gives rise to feelings of victimization and frustration.

Good communication skills are essential in any situation. Make it a habit to employ these skills regularly in your everyday interactions in both home and work environments.

Assertiveness Skills

Assertiveness

Self-assertiveness is defined as "the ability to be comfortably strong-willed with thoughts, feelings, and actions, neither inhibited nor aggressive with actions to the betterment of yourself in your environment." Self-assertiveness has become a major focus for changing stress-related behaviors, particularly in communication skills. Assertiveness skills are behaviors that allow you to feel and express your emotions, opinions, and rights as a human being. Self-assertion is neither a passive attitude that fosters approval and subsequent resentment nor an aggressive style that intimidates others. When you find yourself being taken advantage of, ask yourself, "Was I assertive?"

Assertiveness is one of three styles common to human behavior, positioned between passive and aggressive behaviors. As depicted in the following diagram, behavior styles at either end of the spectrum can promote stress. For example, passive behavior can promote feelings of victimization, while aggressive behavior may indicate unresolved anger.

road to relaxation

Self-Assertiveness Personal Rights*

The following are rights that every person has and should exercise to be assertive:

1. To say "no" and not feel guilty.
2. To change your mind about anything.
3. To take your time to form a response to a comment or question.
4. To ask assistance with instructions or directions.
5. To ask for what you want.
6. To experience and express your feelings.
7. To feel positive about yourself under any conditions.

8. To make mistakes without feeling embarrassed or guilty.
9. To own your own opinions and convictions.
10. To protest unfair treatment or criticism.
11. To be recognized for your significant achievements and contributions.

* Davis, M., Eshelman, E., and McKay, M. The Relaxation and Stress Reduction Workbook. New Harbinger Publications, Inc., Oakland, CA: 1991.

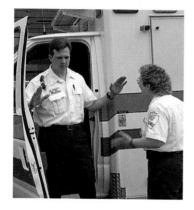

Being assertive means learning how to say "no" comfortably and diplomatically.

Employing Assertive Skills

To change a negative behavior, you must first be aware that what you are doing is undesirable and might in fact be promoting stress. Once you become aware *and* have the desire to change this behavior, you can adopt an alternative behavior. Workshops on assertiveness training teach several skills that you can use to reduce potentially stressful encounters and build self-esteem.

1. *Learn to say no:* Assertiveness training teaches you to say "no" without feeling guilty and worrying that you are hurting the other person's feelings when you cannot afford to take on additional responsibilities. This skill teaches you that you have the right to refuse a request without harboring feelings of guilt and resentment.

2. *Learn to use "I" statements:* The use of "I" statements encourages you to claim ownership of your thoughts, feelings, opinions, perceptions, and beliefs. Assertiveness training encourages you to feel comfortable expressing your feelings and opinions using "I" statements (e.g., "I feel angry about ..." or "I perceive what you said to me to be incorrect"). A cautionary note: "I" statements are important in building self-esteem, but "we" statements are equally important for team building.

3. *Use eye contact:* The lack of eye contact during interpersonal communication is perceived by others as either dishonesty or insecurity about the message. Eye contact is often difficult when you express your feelings toward someone else and fear rejection. Assertiveness training encourages you to use eye contact while expressing your thoughts, feelings, and opinions to others. Practice making eye contact by starting with short time intervals (1 to 2 seconds) and progressing up to 8- to 10-second periods. But remember, just as poor eye contact communicates a lack of confidence, staring (prolonged eye contact) is perceived to be a violation of personal space and should be avoided.

4. *Use assertive body language:* How you stand and position your arms, legs, and body weight can either reinforce your message or detract from it. In addition to eye contact and a reassuring tone of voice, your posture and head position unconsciously reveal how you really feel about the messages you are communicating. When you talk to someone, your posture should

be straight, chin up, with your body weight equally distributed between both legs and your center of gravity maintained directly above your feet.

5. *Practice peaceful disagreement:* When opinions and facts are voiced peacefully so that all perspectives can be considered in a decision-making process, then disagreement is considered healthy. This skill allows you to become comfortable with "peaceful confrontation." Use this skill when you think that you need to express your opposing view and let your voice be heard.

6. *Avoid manipulation:* When you assert yourself, you might find that others, in an effort to control the situation, purposely try to block your efforts to resolve the issue at hand. Manipulation can come in the form of intimidation, content substitution, personal attacks, or avoidance. Be careful not to allow others to derail your assertiveness with *their* style of manipulation.

7. *Respond rather than react:* A reaction is a reflex based upon emotional thoughts. A response, by contrast, is a thought-out strategy to deal with a situation. Too often, reactions replace responses. Take the time to think before speaking or acting on a situation. Respond to a situation by developing an appropriate response to the situation at hand and using it.

Conflict Resolution Skills

Even with effective communication skills and the best intentions, there is an abundance of room for misunderstanding and conflict, at work or at home. Ideally, conflicts are best handled when they are resolved right away; however, this is not always possible, such as when a command supervisor instructs you to use a particular procedure you disagree with. Usually, you need some time to organize your thoughts to resolve a conflict effectively. Regardless, the sooner you respond to a conflict, the better.

Several management styles are used to deal with conflict. Not all styles are beneficial, though; some may actually exacerbate the situation. Although not all conflicts will elicit the same response, it is important to recognize your dominant style and make changes where necessary. Focus on the effective styles and practice using these when conflicts arise at work.

1. *Withdrawal (negative):* Withdrawal can be defined as either a physical or a psychological removal from the problem. Walking out of a room, taking a detour to your office, or remaining silent in the midst of a conversation are examples of withdrawal or avoidance. Typically, withdrawal is regarded as an immature behavior and therefore a negative conflict management style because a physical or verbal absence never resolves anything.

2. *Surrender (negative):* Like withdrawal, surrender is a type of avoidance that people use to appease fellow workers, family, peers, and specifically close friends for fear of rejection and damaging relationships. Surrendering to the will of others by constantly giving in deflates self-esteem. This style of conflict management often generates feelings of self-victimization.

3. *Hostile aggression (negative):* Verbal aggression and underhanded tactics are often used to intimidate and manipulate others. Aggressive behavior will not resolve any conflict and often increases resentment.

4. *Persuasion (positive):* Persuasion is defined as an attempt to alter another person's attitude or behavior. Persuasion may include the use of reason, emotional awareness, or motivation to get a point across. When used tactfully, persuasion opens new lines of thinking, which can then be tools to resolve issues and promote mutual agreement.

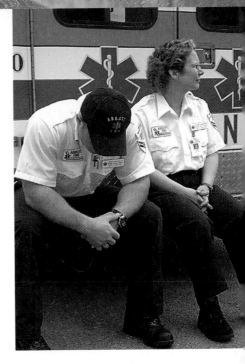

Body language can be more revealing than the spoken word; people are more likely to trust body language than verbal communication when the two differ.

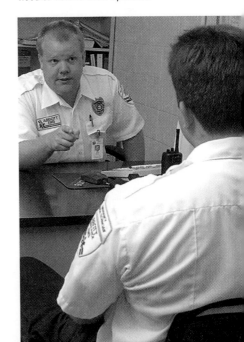

Conflicts often arise when expectations are unmet or people feel the need to defend their opinions.

5. *Open dialogue (positive):* Open dialogue is a verbal exchange of opinions, attitudes, facts, and perceptions by all the people involved. During the dialogue process, discussions center on the costs and benefits involving the steps to creative problem solving. Compromise plays an important role in the dialogue process so that a decision is made that is acceptable to everyone.

Developing Support Networks

A strong social network is now considered a crucial factor in dealing with stress. Having good friends to count on in times of need is a true blessing and can help to buffer the effects of stress.

When factors contributing to the longevity and quality of life of today's elderly are evaluated, one characteristic repeatedly surfaces, friends. Proper diet, regular exercise, adequate sleep, not smoking, low blood pressure, and moderate alcohol consumption are no longer considered the sole essential qualities for living a long and healthy life. A strong network of friends has been consistently shown to be an essential criterion in the quality-of-life equation. Individuals who have a strong support group and feel a healthy connectedness to their family and friends have a better physical and emotional tolerance to stress than those who do not. This has been called the "buffer theory," because in times of need, close friends tend to buffer the ill effects of stress by helping to absorb some of the tension. This aspect of connectedness becomes very important in the work environment. Disgruntled employees who take revenge on managers and co-workers often feel disconnected and alienated from their fellow workers. The message to everyone in today's workforce is twofold:

1. At the worksite, reframe your attitudes and change your behaviors from a competitive nature to a cooperative one. Display a greater sense of acceptance, respect, and tolerance toward co-workers, whatever their gender, race, management position, political persuasion, or differing personal characteristics.

2. Don't spread yourself too thin. Rather than trying to maintain strong friendships with many acquaintances, choose a close handful of friends, both within and outside your family, as your support group. Spend time developing the relationships within your support group.

There is no one-size-fits-all coping technique for stress. Rather, there are a host of coping techniques which when used separately or combined serve as an effective buffer against the stress and strain of personal and professional demands. Coping skills help change threatening perceptions to moments of opportunities and begin resolving the cause of the problem through awareness and acceptance. Coping skills begin in the mind, but the body benefits as well.

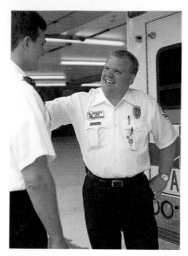

The sooner you can resolve a conflict, the better for all involved.

Having a strong circle of friends tends to buffer the ill effects of stress, making your social support group an essential part of your health.

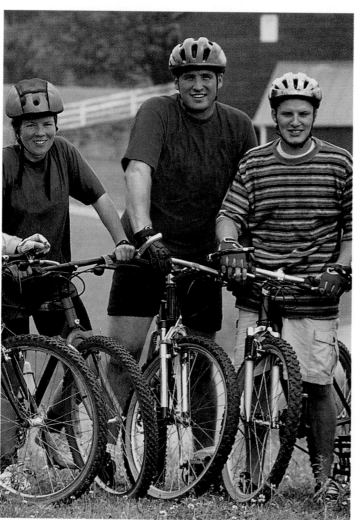

stress | strategies

Exercise ①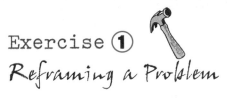
Reframing a Problem

1. Describe a work-related problem that you are currently facing. Explain why you see this as a problem or issue.

2. Describe your feelings about the situation (e.g., anger or fear).

3. Reframe the problem so that it is presented as a challenge rather than a threat.

4. Try reframing the problem again from a third-person perspective.

The dragon is a universal symbol of the unknown. Mapmakers used the dragon to signify unknown territory. People who did not understand the symbol assumed a literal meaning and believed that there were dragons in the waters. Learn to confront your stressors.

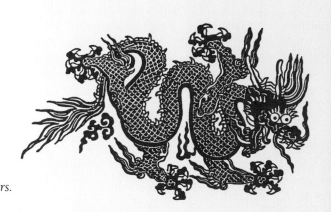

Exercise ②
Creating Solutions

This format may be helpful in writing about a problem.

1. Description of the problem:

2. Generation of ideas (think of at least two viable possibilities):

3. Idea selection and refinement:

4. Idea implementation:

5 Evaluation and analysis of action:

Using this format, write your responses to these two hypothetical problems. Then try the same format with a problem that you have. You might want to refer to the problem you chose in Exercise 1.

Problem 1: As a first responder, you arrive at an accident scene to find a car turned on its side with three people inside: two unconscious and one screaming.

Problem 2: Twenty vials of anthrax have been opened at half-time during a college basketball game. The dispatcher relays a message that there is an emergency on campus. Hundreds of people are sick.

Exercise ③

Expressing It Without Words

Many thoughts and emotions are hard to express in words. Not always, but often, a visual picture that is rich in color, texture, and style can best describe feelings. Art therapy is used in many settings (hospitals, prisons, stress management classes, wellness programs) to help individuals learn to express themselves and their thoughts and feelings visually in a way that words cannot adequately manage. Often, drawings can communicate thoughts from the unconscious that the conscious mind can then begin to decipher and understand, giving a more honest picture of the real you. For example, the colors that are used and the proportions of objects or people can connote specific moods or personal meaning. Exploring thoughts, memories, and feelings from the right side of the brain can often lead to a clearer understanding of their origins and perhaps what they represent. Illustrations, when combined with a narrative, can also be used to enhance memories of journal entries from traumatic events. Art therapy can provide a catharsis, a release of pent-up emotional thoughts and feelings that are begging to be set free.

You don't have to be an artist. You need only crayons, colored pencils, paint, or pastels, some paper, and a desire to illustrate what's on your mind to paper. No one is going to look at what you've done, no one is going to analyze or judge it, nor should you when you complete the picture you have started. For this reason, there is no need to feel inhibited. It doesn't matter whether you produce stick figures or create at the level of Rembrandt or Renoir.

Draw a representation of your feelings evoked from the latest casualty rescue, or draw the rescue itself. This is an idea used in art therapy classes. It is only a suggestion. Feel free to augment it in any way that you feel most comfortable.

Exercise ④
Writing About It

Into each life, a little rain must fall, but sometimes, it seems there's a devastating flood. Broken bones, the death of a close friend or loved one, and child abuse are just a handful of life's many tragedies. "Tragedy," it is said, "keeps a person humble." But it can also leave physical, mental, emotional, and spiritual scars that may take a lifetime to heal. Times like these are often referred to as "the dark night of the soul." Reactions may vary, but nervous talking often occurs immediately after a tragedy.

This is one of the initial manifestations of grief. This stage is often followed by withdrawal and eventually a slow reemergence into society. Traumatic experiences from years ago can also affect your outlook and behaviors on several issues, often unknowingly. EMS personnel who worked at the Oklahoma City Bombing found journal writing to be an excellent therapy to deal with the stress of the mass casualty incident. If you have been spared a personal tragedy, consider yourself lucky. If you have experienced an event of this nature and wish to recount it here, feel free to do so. Peace.

Exercise ⑤
Delving into Dreams

Everyone dreams, although remembering them is not always easy. But there are occasions when a certain dream returns over the course of months, or even years. "Recurring dreams," as they are commonly called, might have only a short run on the mind's silver screen, or they might last throughout the course of a lifetime. These dreams, perhaps foggy in detail, surface occasionally in the conscious state, and the story they tell is all too familiar.

It is commonly believed that recurring dreams symbolize a hidden insecurity or a stressful event that has yet to be resolved. They don't have resolved endings. While there is much to the dream state that is still unknown, dreams are believed to be images that the unconscious mind creates to communicate to the conscious mind. This form of communication is not a one-way street. Messages can be sent to the unconscious mind in a normal waking state as well.

Through the use of mental imagery, you can script the final scenes of a recurring dream to give it a happy ending. What seems to be the final scene of a dream is actually the beginning of the resolution process, as in this true story:

Once there was a young boy who had an afternoon paper route. One day while he was delivering papers, a large, black German shepherd jumped out of the bushes and attacked the boy. The owner called the dog back, but not before the dog drew blood. As the boy grew into adulthood, his love for dogs never diminished, but several times a year, he awoke in a sweat from a recurring dream.

The Dream: *"It's dark and I'm walking through the woods at night. Out from behind one of the trees comes this huge black dog. All I can see are his teeth and hear his bark. I try to yell for help, but nothing comes out of my throat. Just as he lunges for me, I awake in a panic."*

With a little thought and imagination, the young man drafted a final scene to bring closure to this dream story.

Final Scene: *"I am walking through the woods at night with a flashlight, a bone, and a can of mace. This time when the dog lunges at me, I shine the light in his eyes and spray mace in his face. He whines and whines, and then I tell him to sit. He obeys. I put the bone by his nose, and he looks at me inquisitively. Then he licks the bone and starts to bite into it. I begin to walk away, and the dog gets up to follow, bone in mouth. I stop and look back, and he stops. He wags his tail. The sky grows light as the sun begins to rise, and the black night fades into pink and orange clouds. As I walk back to my house, I see the dog take his new find down the street. I open the door and walk upstairs and crawl back into bed."* It has been five years, and this individual has never had this dream again.

Ultimately, you create your dreams. You are the writer, director, producer, and actor of your dreams. Although drafting a final scene is no guarantee of resolution for the issues that produce recurring dreams, it is a great starting point toward the resolution process, a time for reflection that might open up the channels of communication between the conscious mind and the unconscious mind. Is there a recurring dream that you have that needs a final scene to be complete? Write out your recurring dream and give it a final scene.

Exercise ⑥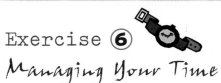
Managing Your Time

Time Robbers

List five things that steal or waste time away from your day:

1.

2.

3.

4.

5.

ABC RANK ORDER METHOD OF TIME MANAGEMENT

Directions: Make a list of tasks and responsibilities. Then place in Column A all the things that must get done as soon as possible. In Column C, list all the things that you would like to do, but that are not essential (watching TV). In Column B, put everything else.

A MUST DO	B SHOULD DO	C WANT TO DO
_____	_____	_____
_____	_____	_____
_____	_____	_____
_____	_____	_____

Exercise ⑦
Asserting Yourself

This is an exercise to increase your awareness of your own assertiveness skills. The example is a hypothetical circumstance that could produce feelings of anger, fear, and potential victimization. Please write your initial response in the space provided, followed by a more assertive response if needed. Then think of a situation in your own life and follow the same procedure.

Situation 1:

A squad member tells you that he has a wedding to go to next week and wants to know whether you can cover his shift while he's away.

Initial Reaction:

Assertive Response:

Situation 2:

_____

_____

Initial Reaction:

Assertive Response:

Exercise ⑧

Identifying Your Support Network

Take a moment to make an inventory of your support network and what you can do to strengthen your ties with individuals who provide you with support.

1. List three people at work with whom you feel comfortable enough to trust and confide in about your present work situation.

   a.

   b.

   c.

2. List three people *outside* your family with whom you spend quality time on a regular basis.

   a.

   b.

   c.

3. Make a list of three interests or activities in which you participate outside of work and home.

   a.

   b.

   c.

4. Locate two groups of people in your area who share a similar interest. Try to connect with them once or twice a month.

   a.

   b.

5. Have you been out of touch with anyone you've listed? Could you contact and meet with them to solidify your friendship bonds?

   a.

   b.

   c.

Relaxation Techniques

Sandra, a dispatcher in Washington, D.C., goes for walks on her lunch break. She says it's not for the fresh air, it's for the peace of mind.

When Zach comes home from the station, the TV goes off, the stereo goes on, and instrumental music fills the house for the next few hours. Donna treats herself to a massage once a month, a practice she started after her first sports massage after the Ironman Triathlon in Hawaii. Keith learned deep breathing with his wife in a Lamaze course, and he has continued to use the same technique in every critical incident he has been involved in. For these people and others like them, relaxation techniques are not just a theoretical concept; they are a way of life.

You are always absorbing messages from your five senses: sight, sound, smell, taste, and touch. Information picked up through one or more of these senses is continually sent to the brain. If a message is considered a threat, an alarm sounds and the body prepares to move as a means of survival. In order to relax from any sort of panicked response and return the body to a state of calmness or *homeostasis*, something must be done to turn down the amount of stimulation that the senses take in. In other words, the five senses must be *deactivated* or *reprogrammed*, if only temporarily, to give the body a new signal to calm down. The primary purpose of relaxation techniques is to interrupt the stress response, specifically through the nervous and hormonal systems. Ultimately, relaxation techniques help to reduce the physical symptoms of stress when the body works overtime to keep up with everyday issues, hassles, and worries.

Unfortunately, relaxation techniques are not a form of magic. What provides a calming effect for one person might offer nothing but added frustration for another. The ability to relax depends largely on the individual. In addition, no one technique is effective for all people in all circumstances. Becoming familiar with several techniques lets you pick one or two that you like to make your body more resistant to the effects of stress. Relaxation techniques are skills just like intubating a patient or throwing a strike, and you need to practice them regularly to get the full benefits. Regardless of which technique you choose, you should practice some form of relaxation every day for about 20 to 30 minutes. Used regularly, relaxation skills provide you with the best defense against the hazards of the stressful wear and tear on your body and promote a greater sense of well-being.

Because the mind-body connection is so strong, you might find that relaxation techniques not only create a physical calming effect, they also seem to calm the mind. For this reason, activities such as jogging, meditation, and listening to music can help you to cope with stress as well. One common misconception is that relaxation is the same thing as sleep. Nothing could be farther from the truth.

> **T**hat the birds fly overhead, this you cannot stop. That they build a nest in your hair, this you can prevent.
>
> **Ancient Chinese proverb**

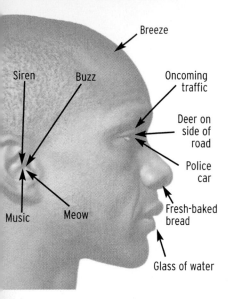

Breeze

Siren   Buzz

Oncoming traffic

Deer on side of road

Police car

Fresh-baked bread

Music   Meow

Glass of water

The five senses gather information. Relaxation techniques are used to deactivate the sensory organs and give the body a chance to return to a resting state.

> **Let the air breathe for you.**
> Emitt Miller, M.D.

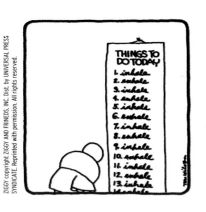

Relaxation techniques might make you sleep better, but sleeping should not be used instead of proper relaxation skills.

The origins of these relaxation techniques span many continents and cultures over several thousands of years. For example, from Asia come the techniques of diaphragmatic breathing, yoga, meditation, massage therapy, and tai chi. Several aspects of these are now combined with many Western techniques such as mental imagery, autogenic training, music therapy, and physical exercise. Once you feel confident in performing these skills, you will find that some are better suited for dealing with stress immediately, while other methods are more useful at either the beginning or the end of the day. This section will highlight physical relaxation techniques such as diaphragmatic breathing, progressive muscular relaxation, autogenic training, physical exercise, and music therapy, and mental relaxation techniques such as meditation and mental imagery.

Physical Relaxation Techniques

StressLess
EMS

www.StressLessEMS.com

Diaphragmatic Breathing

Diaphragmatic breathing is by far the easiest relaxation technique to learn and practice. It is easy because breathing is a normal action, done without thought or hesitation. This technique can be done anywhere, at any time. Diaphragmatic breathing is the quintessential deep sigh of relief. In its simplest form, diaphragmatic breathing is slow, conscious "deep breathing." You probably take a big breath when you are regrouping your thoughts, trying to gain composure, or directing your energies for a challenging task. Most people are accustomed to breathing with the upper chest (stop for a moment and pay attention to how you breathe). When fast asleep without the influence of the conscious mind, everyone reverts back to a more natural breathing posture, with greater stomach expansion. Diaphragmatic breathing is different from "normal breathing" because this method specifically involves the *conscious movement* of the lower abdomen or belly area. For EMS professionals who are involved in critical care of any kind, diaphragmatic breathing is perhaps the best relaxation technique that can be done on-site. It can help you keep calm in the midst of acute stress as well as during less tense situations.

The Art of Relaxed Breathing

Under normal resting conditions, you breathe approximately 14 to 16 times per minute. When you become panicked, your breath quickens and becomes more shallow, with stronger muscular contraction of the upper chest. When the upper chest expands, neural stimulation is increased, and your vital signs (heart rate, blood pressure) begin to rise. During heavy aerobic exercise, you breathe up to 60 times per minute because your body needs more oxygen. When you are relaxed, your body's metabolism is much slower, allowing for a slower, deeper breathing cycle. When you learn to modify your breathing style (with an emphasis on diaphragmatic breathing), you may be able to comfortably reduce the number of breaths to as low as 3 to 6 breaths per minute.

The practice of diaphragmatic breathing is as old as the ancient exercises of yoga and tai chi. It is now a part of virtually every relaxation technique. As a relaxation technique, diaphragmatic breathing focuses on just one body sensation: feeling air slowly pass through your nose or mouth down into your lungs and return via the same pathway, to the exclusion of all other sensory stimulation.

Body Position

To gain the most benefit, learn this technique in a comfortable position, either in a relaxed sitting position or lying on your back with your eyes closed. Loosen any constrictive clothing around your neck and waist. As you practice this technique, place your hands over your stomach and feel its rise and fall with each breath. Once you mastered this skill, you can do diaphragmatic breathing practically anywhere, while driving your car, participating in a job performance review, waiting in line, or giving a professional presentation.

Concentration and Awareness

Like all relaxation techniques, diaphragmatic breathing requires your undivided attention. Concentration can be easily interrupted by both external noises (a ringing phone) and internal thoughts ("Am I doing this right?"). When possible, take steps to minimize external interruptions by finding a nice, quiet place to practice. When first learning this and other techniques that require total concentration, you will notice that sometimes your mind will begin to wander. This is normal. If you find that your mind becomes preoccupied with other thoughts, just allow them to fade away and then refocus your attention on your breathing. You could imagine these interrupting thoughts escaping through your mouth as you exhale or you can keep a piece of paper and pen beside you and write down these thoughts as they appear, just to get them out of your head.

Breathing

Diaphragmatic breathing requires a conscious decision to focus your attention solely on your breathing. Imagine following the flow of air as it enters your body, goes to its destination in the lower portion of your lungs, and moves back out again. You may want to say to yourself, *"I feel the air coming into my nose or mouth and down into my lungs, and I feel my stomach rise and fall as I exhale the air, feeling it leave my lungs, throat, and nasal cavity"* with each breath.

Focus on the four distinct phases of each breath:

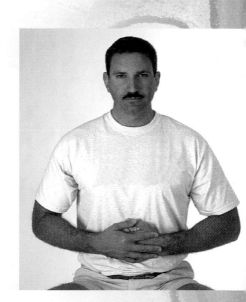

As you practice diaphragmatic breathing, place your hands on your stomach to feel it rise and fall with each breath.

- *Phase I:* The inspiration, taking the air into your lungs through your nose or mouth.

- *Phase II:* A very slight pause before exhaling the air out of your lungs.

- *Phase III:* The exhalation, releasing the air from your lungs and back out through the passage by which it entered.

- *Phase IV:* A very slight pause after exhalation before beginning the next inhalation.

You can notice these phases when you exaggerate the breathing cycle by taking a very slow and comfortable deep breath. As you do this, try to identify each phase as it occurs. Remember, do not hold your breath at any time. Rather, learn to regulate your breathing by controlling the pace of each phase in the breathing cycle. *Diaphragmatic breathing is not the same as hyperventilation.* It is comfortably slow, deep, and relaxed. You will feel most relaxed during the third phase, the exhalation phase, when the chest and stomach areas relax and a calming effect permeates throughout your whole body. It requires no effort whatsoever. As you focus on your breathing, feel how relaxed your whole body becomes during the exhalation phase, especially your chest, shoulders, and stomach region. With practice, this relaxation will spread throughout your whole body.

> **Relaxation is the direct negative of nervous excitement. It is the absence of nerve-muscle impulse.**
> Edmund Jacobson, M.D.

Facial stretch.

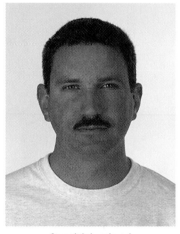

Completely relaxed

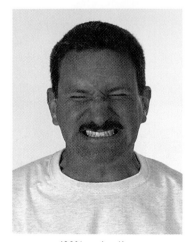

100% contraction

Visualization

The use of imagery with diaphragmatic breathing can be very powerful. Many images can be combined with this breathing technique. Exercise 1 at the end of this chapter may help you with this technique.

Progressive Muscular Relaxation

Your body's muscles respond to perceived threats with neural tension, or a state of contraction. As a result, muscular tension is believed to be the most common symptom of stress. Although muscular tension does not send people to hospital emergency rooms like other stress-related disorders, the overall effect can result in much stiffness, pain, and discomfort due to muscular imbalance. In extreme cases, muscular tension can cause postural abnormalities and misalignment as well as joint instability. Muscle tension can appear as tension headaches, neck stiffness, lower back pain, stomach cramps, and some forms of temporomandibular joint dysfunction (TMJ).

Often, muscle tension can occur while you sleep from thoughts in the unconscious mind. Experts note that joint stiffness and even damaged connective tissue in the jaw, neck, shoulders, and lower back can result from muscle tension during sleep. Developed by Dr. Edward Jacobson over 60 years ago, Progressive Muscular Relaxation (PMR) is a technique specifically designed to consciously help reduce muscle tension. You do this by first becoming consciously aware of your muscle tension levels and then reducing the level of tension through relaxation. Currently, PMR therapy is used to help relieve several stress-related symptoms, including insomnia, hypertension, headaches, lower back pain, and TMJ. This technique, perhaps more than any other, illustrates the importance of intercepting the stress response by consciously trying to decrease muscle tension.

There are some cautions to be noted if you use this technique. Isometric muscle tension, used during the contraction phases of PMR, increases both systolic and diastolic blood pressure even with contractions of short duration. Individuals who have hypertension (elevated systolic and/or diastolic blood pressure) *should not* use this technique, because it will certainly aggravate this condition.

Body Position

PMR can be performed in a comfortable sitting position; however, the best position to first learn and practice this method is lying comfortably on a carpeted floor. Your arms should rest naturally by each side with your palms facing upward. Loosen any tight clothing around your neck and waist and remove any jewelry (such as wristwatch and bracelets), as well as eyeglasses or contact lenses before you begin.

Breathing

The breathing technique in PMR is quite simple. Inhale as you contract the muscles, and then exhale as you release the tension. Tension release is coordinated with the release of air in the lungs, and the relaxation of the diaphragm allows for a deeper sense of total relaxation throughout the entire body.

Ambiance

If necessary, adjust the room temperature to a mild environment. A cool environment can produce unwanted muscle tension expressed as shivering. Once you are proficient in the technique, you can do PMR anywhere: sitting in traffic, standing in line, or lying in bed trying to fall asleep. Practice this technique every day to feel the effects immediately.

Muscle Contractions

The best way to do PMR is to tighten and relax each muscle group in the body systematically, one muscle group at a time. Contract the muscle group at 100% intensity (all out) for 5 seconds, then relax for 45 seconds. Next, contract the muscle group at 50% intensity (half the strength of the initial contraction) for 5 seconds, then relax for 45 seconds. Finally, contract the muscle group for 5% intensity (a slight twinge), then relax for 45 seconds before moving to the next muscle group. In the release phase, take a comfortably deep breath and feel a sense of relaxation in the muscle group that was previously tensed. Compare this sensation with how the muscle felt when it was contracted. Try the following order of muscle groups: face (included the eyes and brow), jaw, neck, shoulders, upper chest, forearms, hands, stomach, quadriceps, calves, and feet. Remember that only one muscle group should be contracted at a time, leaving all other muscle groups relaxed. It might seem hard at first not to involve surrounding muscles, but this will come with practice.

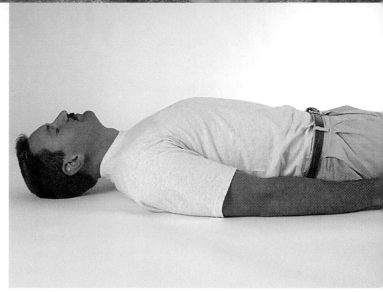

The supine position is ideal for learning PMR.

Progressive Muscular Relaxation Suggestions

When you are finished with the technique, lie still on the floor or sit still in your chair for a few minutes and pay attention to all physical sensations. Enjoy the full sense of relaxation. Then begin to focus your thoughts on your current surroundings. By feeling the different degrees of muscle contraction, you might find that you become more aware of your own muscle tension levels in the course of a day and then become able to adjust them through tension release.

The advantage of PMR is its direct approach to reduce muscle tension by contracting and relaxing specific muscle groups. The relaxation effect becomes evident when you compare the state of tension with relaxation. In whole or part, this technique is easy to learn and practice in a variety of settings: at the station while on break, in transport to the scene of an accident, or at home. You can use PMR in the morning as a prevention technique or in the evening to help release tension that accumulated in the course of a stressful day. Exercise 2 at the end of this chapter may help you with this technique.

Autogenic Training

The word "autogenic" means self-regulation or self-generation. It can also refer to an action that is self-produced. The term "autogenic training" implies that you have the conscious ability to actually control various body functions such as heart rate, blood pressure, and blood flow. This is a novel concept for many Western cultures because for centuries, specific body functions were thought to operate independently of self-directed thoughts. Research over the last two decades has proved differently. By consciously redirecting your body's responses with your own suggestions, you can help to negate the harmful effects of stress through the powerful mind-body connection. In fact, you can learn how to step in and take over from the automatic pilot of your nervous system whenever you want to override the stress response to nonphysical threats.

The premise of autogenic training is to learn how to redirect the mind with suggestions so that you can override the stress response when physical arousal is not the appropriate reaction. The major autogenic suggestion that you give to yourself

> **Open your mind to the power of self-suggestion.**
> Johannes Schultz

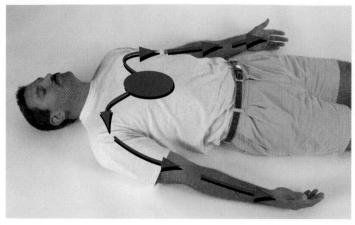

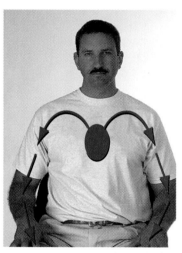

There are two suggested body positions for practicing autogenic training. The preferred method is a supine position on a comfortable floor surface. If this is not possible, then a sitting position will do fine. Once you are proficient in this technique, you can do it in any position.

is to allow various body regions (the arms, hands, legs, and feet) to become warm and heavy. This sensation of warmth and heaviness, due to a shift of blood flow from the body's center to the desired area, acts like an internal massage, soothing and relaxing the surrounding muscles. Unlike diaphragmatic breathing, which can be done just about anywhere, this relaxation technique is best performed with little or no distraction. It could be done during lulls at the station, but it's not generally a technique to use in the field. (However, this technique has been used for some patients in surgery to reduce bleeding, with significant results!)

The principles of autogenic training can be learned quite quickly. The short-term effects are often experienced immediately; however, it might take a few weeks of practice to feel the cumulative effects. When you are learning and practicing autogenic training, practice once a day for 15 minutes at a time.

Body Position

The best position for this technique is lying down on your back on a carpeted floor or bed with your arms by your sides, palms facing up, and legs straight with your heels resting evenly on the surface. Thin pillows or cushions may be used behind the head and knees for support as long as the body remains comfortable with your spine straight. If circumstances do not permit you to lie down, sit straight up in a chair. While seated, keep your head aligned over your body with your arms either on your lap or supported by the frame of the chair. Remove watches, rings, necklaces, and chains and loosen any restrictive clothing. Perhaps most important, try not to eat a big meal beforehand, because food in your stomach will make this technique less effective.

Concentration and Awareness

Allow yourself to become open to suggestion and adopt a passive, not defensive, frame of mind. Concentrate on the here and now, specifically the present state of your body. When you first try autogenic training, you might find your mind drifting toward what seem like more important thoughts. If you find other thoughts competing for your attention, politely acknowledge them and then focus your mind back on your body awareness. With continued practice, your ability to concentrate will improve.

Phases of Autogenic Training

The four phases of autogenic training include a feeling of *heaviness,* a feeling of *warmth,* a *calmness of the heart,* and a *calmness of breathing.* Dedicate between three and four minutes to each phase. Tell yourself that your arms, legs, hands and feet feel heavy, then tell yourself that your arms, legs, hands, and feet feel warm. Next, tell yourself that your heartbeat is slow and calm. Finally, tell yourself that your breathing is relaxed and your entire body feels calm and comfortable. The entire progression of phases should take approximately 15 minutes. When you are done, remain in the same position for a few moments and try to place this feeling of relaxation into your memory bank so that you can recall it at times when you feel stressed.

Originally, autogenic training was used to relax just the arms and hands, but it can relax all body regions. The autogenic technique is as portable as the thoughts that create it. You can use it at home, at work, or anywhere.

At the worksite, you may be able to take short, periodic autogenic breaks in the course of a busy day as a preventive approach to the cumulative effects of the stress response. Exercise 3 at the end of this chapter may help you with this technique.

> **A sound mind in a sound body.**
> Ancient Greek Proverb

Physical Exercise and Nutrition

For many people, physical exercise is a popular and effective way to reduce stress. Quite literally, it allows you to express the fight or flight response. Although exercise actually triggers the stress response, when you stop exercising, the body returns to a greater state of calmness than before you began, a condition called "parasympathetic rebound." For a person who is well conditioned, not only is the rate of return quicker, but the degree of physical calmness is greater than before exercise was started. It seems that the body's natural response, when confronted with stress, is to be active, which is why regular exercise is so beneficial.

In the past 30 years, since the recognition of coronary heart disease and its associated risk factors as North America's number one cause of death, the effects of physical exercise on the human body have been studied intensely. The overwhelming conclusion is that physical exercise is a virtual necessity to maintain the proper functions of the body's vital organs. Just as the body requires physical calmness, it equally demands physical exercise. There must be a balance between physical arousal (activity) and physical calmness (rest) to achieve optimal wellness.

Physical exercise serves as an effective relaxation technique because it releases the same stress hormones needed for the fight or flight response and uses them for their intended metabolic purpose. Epinephrine and norepinephrine work to increase heart rate and blood pressure, promote sweating, and quicken your breathing cycle. Cortisol allows for the mobilization of glucose and free fatty acids into the blood for energy. Aldosterone increases blood pressure to get blood and oxygen to the extremities for rapid movement. It seems that physical exercise actually helps build an immunity to stress and strengthens the body's vital organs. Exercise physiologists have observed many positive adaptations of the cardiovascular, musculoskeletal, and immune systems when people exercise regularly. The body, it seems, can adapt to the good stress of exercise as well as bad stress of emotional turmoil.

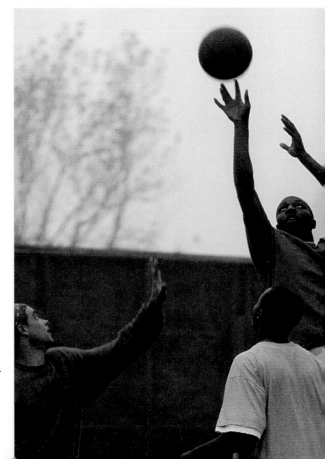

Regular exercise is one of the most popular and effective means to reduce physical stress.

Types of Physical Exercise

Although there are many types of exercise, including swimming, weight lifting, and golf, all physical activity falls into two categories:

1. *Anaerobic exercise:* Exercise that involves intense bursts of energy for short amounts of time (seconds to minutes). Weight lifting, sprints, and some calisthenics are the most common examples of this type of activity. Anaerobic exercise focuses on muscular strength and power.

2. *Aerobic exercise:* Aerobic exercise or cardiovascular endurance activities are described as "rhythmic" or "continuous" in nature. Aerobic work involves moderate intensity for an extended period of time (over 20 minutes). Intensity is typically measured by heart rate (beats per minute). Running, swimming, cycling, cross-country skiing, rhythmic dancing, and walking are examples of aerobic activity.

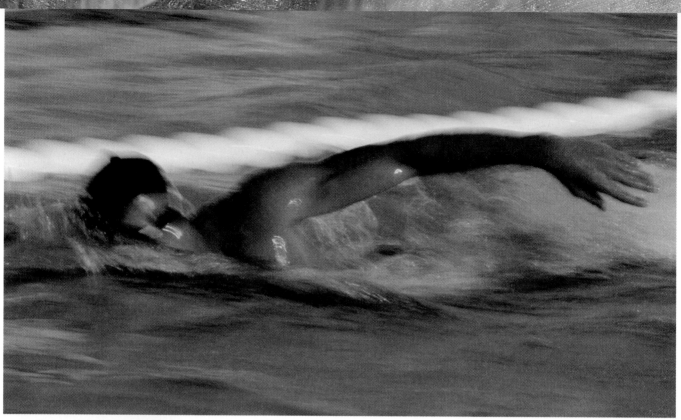

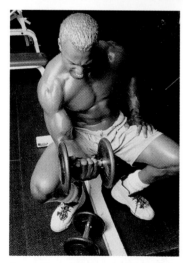

Types of exercises vary by the specific energy system used. Short bursts of activity (weight training) are considered anaerobic, whereas prolonged rhythmical exercises (swimming, walking, or jogging) are considered aerobic in nature.

Aerobic exercise helps reduce the risk of heart disease by modifying several coronary risk factors in the following ways:

1. Reducing elevated blood pressure.

2. Decreasing resting heart rate.

3. Reducing cholesterol, specifically low-density lipoproteins (LDLs).

4. Significantly decreasing percent of body fat.

5. Increasing physical activity.

6. Decreasing physical arousal due to acute and chronic stress.

The Physiological Effects of Physical Exercise

A single aerobic exercise workout "burns off" stress hormones, using them for their intended metabolic function. Because these stress hormones are used on a regular

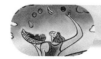

help your health

Feel the Burn!

The caloric equivalent (calories burned) during a 30-minute period for a person weighing approximately 143 pounds vary depending on the activity, as shown:

Brisk walking	230 cal	Golf	129 cal
Swimming	249 cal	Racquetball	348 cal
Jogging	400 cal	Aerobic dance	201 cal

basis, the body does *not* release large amounts of stress hormones when feelings of anger or fear surface. In effect, exercise training tends to neutralize physical arousal to nonphysical threats. Furthermore, the long-term effects of exercise produced by at least 6 to 8 weeks of training appear to strengthen the body's vital organs. Exercise conditioning isn't a cure for diseases and illness, nor is it a "fountain of youth." However, athletic conditioning does appear to add to the quality and even the quantity of life.

Theories of Athletic Conditioning

Numerous studies have been conducted to determine the minimal amount of exercise needed to maintain the benefits gained through physical labor. Four key ingredients are necessary to reap the beneficial effects of exercise:

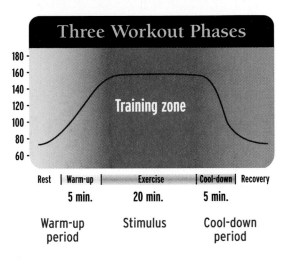

1. *Intensity:* Intensity refers to the challenge (stress) placed on the body in response to the activity. It is often expressed as your target heart rate or target zone: the range of heartbeats during rhythmic exercise calculated to be in the range of 60-80% of maximal intensity. (Achieving your target heart rate is discussed in Exercise 4 at the end of this chapter).

2. *Frequency:* Frequency refers to the number of exercise sessions per week. Three sessions per week are needed to maintain your level of fitness.

3. *Duration:* Duration is the number of minutes per session. The suggested duration is a minimum of 20 to 30 minutes at your target heart rate per exercise session. Exercising less than 20 minutes does not necessarily guarantee the full benefits of endurance exercise.

4. *Mode of exercise:* The mode of exercise is the specific type of activity that you choose to challenge your body. For example, walking, running, and swimming are considered aerobic work and challenge the cardiovascular system adequately, whereas weight training uses the anaerobic energy system and may not effectively challenge the cardiovascular system.

Of the three phases of a workout-warm-up, stimulus, and cool-down-the stimulus phase is when your target heart rate should remain elevated. The more efficient your cardiovascular system, the sooner your heart rate will return to a normal resting level.

Phases of a Workout

There is a formula to follow to ensure a safe workout each time you exercise: a proper warm-up, the stimulus or conditioning period, and a cool-down.

1. *Warm-up period:* The purpose of the warm-up is to slowly increase the heart rate, allowing adequate time for the working muscles to become saturated in oxygen-rich blood. The warm-up period should consist of any activity, such as walking, slow jogging, or calisthenics, at a low intensity. Once your body has warmed up, you can stretch your muscles. Stretching before you exercise may lead to tendon or ligament damage.

2. *Stimulus period:* The stimulus period is the real "meat" of the workout. This is the actual period that conditions the heart, lungs, and muscles. The stimulus period should be a minimum of 20 minutes, regardless of which energy system (aerobic or anaerobic) is used. As you continue past the first 8 weeks of training, you may wish to increase the stimulus period.

3. *Cool-down period:* The purpose of the cool-down period is to decrease the signs and symptoms of the stress response: heart rate, blood pressure, ventilations, and so on. The cool-down phase, a 5- to 10-minute period, should start with a decreased intensity of activity (e.g., from running to jogging to walking) followed by a few moments of stretching.

A good cool-down consists of slowly decreasing your pace of activity to allow the heart rate and blood pressure to return to normal, followed by stretching.

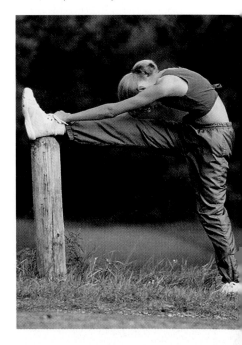

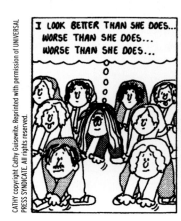
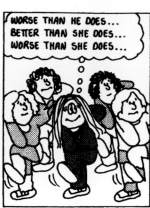
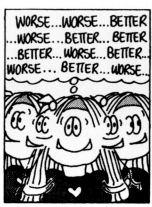
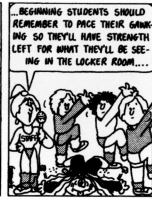

Steps to Initiate a Fitness Training Program

Although physical exercise is one of the best ways to stay healthy, it also poses a threat to your health if not done correctly. Some suggestions to help you avoid injury and burnout include:

1. Set some realistic personal fitness goals for yourself.

2. Start cautiously and progress moderately with your program.
   (If you are over 35 years of age, the American College of Sports Medicine highly recommends that you get a physician's approval before starting an exercise program.)

3. Pick an activity that you really enjoy.

4. Select a time of day to exercise.

5. Exercise in the right clothes and using the right equipment.

6. Initiate an exercise support group to help you stay motivated.

7. Ensure care and prevention of athletic injuries, from blisters and tendonitis to stress fractures and dehydration.

There is no doubt about it. The body needs regular exercise. When you are tired and feel that you don't have the time, that is the time you need it the most. Your body also needs good fuel to burn. To get the best benefits of habitual physical exercise, it must be of the right intensity, frequency, and duration as well as the best mode of exercise. Make it point to get some exercise, even if it is simply going for a brisk 20-minute walk every day.

The Nutrition/Stress Relationship

By and large, when you are stressed, you tend to eat poorly. As a result, your body does not get the essential nutrients it needs, placing even more stressors on your body. Stress also depletes essential nutrients, including a host of vitamins and minerals necessary for optimal functioning and performance. As a result, your health is compromised, and although your body can adapt to some stress in the short term, over time the consequences can be serious.

Many unnatural, toxic substances in processed food today make the "eat a balanced meal" approach to nutrition inadequate for maintaining good health and wellness. The American Cancer Society now states that as much as 60% of cancer is related to diet. The average American diet does not contain adequate amounts of fiber, essential fatty acids, alkaline-based foods, antioxidants, bioflavinoids, and phytonutrients-all essential for good health and optimal performance.

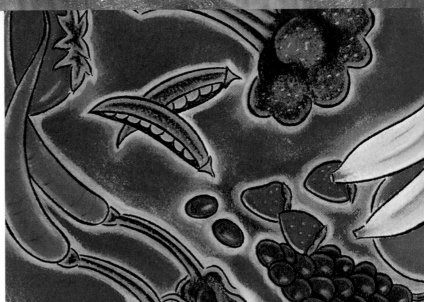

Furthermore, there are several substances that, when consumed, tend to mimic or start the stress response, creating a "Catch-22." Here are some examples:

1. *Caffeine:* Food sources that contain caffeine trigger the stress response, increasing your heart rate. The result is a heightened state of alertness that makes you more susceptible to perceived stress. Caffeine can be found in many foods, including chocolate, coffee, tea, and several beverages.

2. *Sugar:* Excess amounts of simple sugars (found in soda, candy, etc.) tend to deplete vitamin stores, particularly the vitamin B-complex (niacin, thiamin, riboflavin, and B-12). This can lead to fatigue, anxiety, and irritability. In addition, eating large amounts of simple sugars can cause large fluctuations in your blood glucose levels, resulting in pronounced fatigue, headaches, and general irritability.

Prolonged stress can deplete vitamin stores in the body. The best source of vitamins and minerals is natural unprocessed food, including seasonal fruits and vegetables.

3. *Salt:* High sodium intake is associated with high blood pressure, because sodium increases water retention. As water volume increases, blood pressure increases. If this condition persists, it can contribute to hypertension.

4. *Junk food:* Processed food is filled with empty calories (calories that may have some energy component but no nutrition value). As a result, your body becomes malnourished from lack of the essential nutrients and deficient in various vitamins and minerals, including vitamins A, B, C, and E (A, C, and E are antioxidants) and the minerals magnesium, chromium, copper, zinc, iron, and calcium.

Recommendations for Healthy Eating Habits

A few simple changes in your diet can help to minimize your body's arousal to stress and enhance optimal well-being.

1. Eat a well balanced diet, containing the proper amounts of carbohydrates, fats, and proteins.

2. Eat a good breakfast and space meals evenly throughout the day.

3. Avoid or minimize your consumption of caffeine, sugar, and salt.

4. Eat a diet that provides adequate levels of vitamins and minerals that are vulnerable to stress.

 help your health

Typical American Diet		U.S. RDA Suggested Diet	
Carbohydrates:	30-40%	Carbohydrates:	55-70%
Fats:	40-50%	Fats:	20-30%
Proteins:	20-30%	Proteins:	15-20%

5. Be sure to consume the essential fatty acid omega 3 (linolinic acid). This can be found in cold-water fish such as salmon and tuna as well as in flaxseed oil. Balance essential oils omega 3 and 6.

6. Fiber is essential for the prevention of both cancer and coronary heart disease. Most people barely get 5 grams of fiber per day. The World Health Organization recommends 40 to 50 grams.

7. If you take a vitamin supplement, be sure that it is bioavailable (capable of being absorbed into your bloodstream). Many popular brands are made with binders that are not digested and are often excreted. To determine whether your current vitamin brand is bioavailable, place one teaspoon of vinegar in a glass of water and then drop the supplement in. If the pill doesn't dissolve in 15 minutes, find one that does.

8. Minimize your consumption of hydrogenated or partially hydrogenated oils, which are common in many packaged foods because they promote shelf life.

9. Increase your consumption of raw vegetables. Vegetables are a great source of fiber and are rich in phytonutrients, which may help fight the proliferation of cancer cells.

10. Minimize your consumption of artificial food products, including aspartame, a sweetener (now called an excitotoxin) associated with poor cognitive functioning (alertness, mental acuity, headaches, etc.).

Music Therapy

A 1991 survey on relaxation revealed that over 70% of the people questioned preferred to relax by listening to music. Perhaps the proverb "Music soothes the savage beast" has more than a ring of truth to it. Just how music contributes to relaxation is not quite fully understood. Sound is energy made audible. Music is sound appreciated. The laws of physics come into play regarding sympathetic resonance and entrainment (the mutual phase locking of like rhythms). In the simplest terms, it appears that the body's rhythms, from brain waves to heart and muscle waves, can become entrained to the pulsations of musical rhythms. This can promote arousal as well as homeostasis.

Brain lateralization research reveals that instrumental music promotes right brain dominance, often associated with the relaxation response. Therefore, instrumental music, such as classical, jazz, acoustic, new age, can have the greatest relaxation effect. Words or lyrics tend to engage the analytical/judgmental mind and compromise relaxation. The type of instrumental music that works best for you clearly depends on your musical preference. Exercise 6 at the end of this chapter will help you identify this music.

Many stores play music to encourage customers to stay longer and buy more products (and it works). Movie soundtracks create a mood and draw you into the film. Music can excite or relax, and its influence on the nervous system means that music can be used to promote mind-body-spirit homeostasis when the need arises.

Other Relaxation Techniques

Several other physical techniques promote relaxation, some of which you may already use. These include the practice of tai chi (and other martial arts),

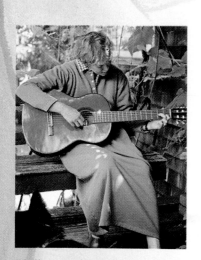

Whether you play music or just listen to it, music has a way of calming the nervous system.

hatha yoga, biofeedback, and body work that incorporates various types of muscle massage, including Swedish massage, sports massage, shiatsu, myofascial release, rolfing, and reflexology, as well as related energy work (e.g., reiki, bioenergy, trigger point therapy, zero point balancing, and therapeutic touch). Muscle tension is the number one symptom of stress. It might not affect your health status immediately, but muscle tension can eventually lead to misalignment to your skeletal structure and connective fascia and a host of related problems. Any form of body work is highly recommended to people who work in the health services professions.

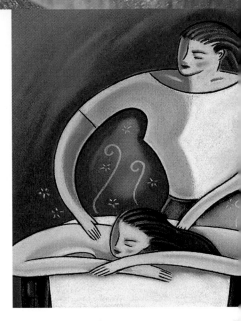

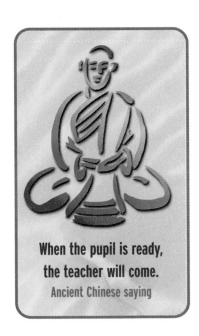

Massage is a welcome relaxation technique to relax stiff, tense muscles caused by stress.

Mental Relaxation

www.StressLessEMS.com

Meditation

Meditation is best described as "an increased concentration and awareness," a process to clear the mind and *live in the present moment.* The practice of meditation is the oldest recognized relaxation technique known to all civilizations. Several components of meditation have been incorporated into virtually every other relaxation technique.

Many studies have been done on the benefits of meditation. Research findings reveal that people who meditate regularly show fewer signs of anxiety; decrease their use of smoking, alcohol, and recreational drugs; demonstrate a greater sense of self-esteem, self-confidence, and self-reliance; and are able to sleep more soundly than people who don't meditate. Today, therapists commonly use meditation as a way to promote psychological well-being. Because meditation has proven to be so effective in lowering the resting heart rate, blood pressure, muscle tension, and other metabolic functions, the American Heart Association now advocates this technique as a way to help prevent coronary heart disease. You may be particularly interested to discover the increased mental acuity that results from the practice of meditation, which is in demand in situations of high-stress performance.

www.StressLessEMS.com

Calming the Mind

Under stress, your mind can become overwhelmed with distractions. Your mind juggles many thoughts, sparked both internally (by memories, feelings, etc.) and externally (by conversations, traffic, radio broadcasts, etc.), all of which compete for attention. As these thoughts accumulate, your mind gets cluttered, your attention span is shortened, and you experience *sensory overload.* Sensory overload is compared to a blackboard filled with unorganized, illegible notes, scribbles, and information. Meditation becomes the eraser to clean the blackboard. When your mind becomes clear of cluttered thoughts, you become more receptive to intuitive insight, new perspectives, and new ways of dealing with your unresolved problems. This is the primary purpose of meditation: increased concentration, which promotes self-awareness.

When the pupil is ready, the teacher will come.
Ancient Chinese saying

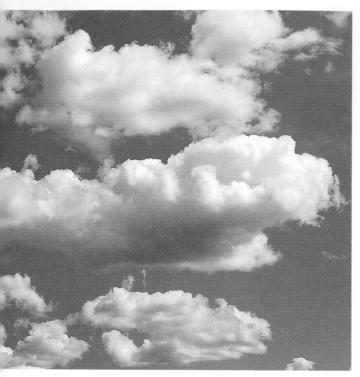

To illustrate the concept of the mind in concrete terms, a cloud metaphor is often used to symbolize your thoughts, feelings, memories, and perceptions. Meditation acts like a wind that blows the clouds away and clears the mind of cluttered thoughts.

Types of Meditation

Eastern philosophy gave rise to two distinct branches of meditation: *exclusive* (restrictive meditation) and *inclusive* (opening-up meditation). Although they vary in style and format, the result is the same: a cleansing of the mind that leads to a sensation that can best be described as "inner peace."

Exclusive Meditation: Exclusive meditation (also known as *concentration meditation*) asks that you restrict your attention to a single thought. This single thought becomes a device to rid all other thoughts from your mind. A single thought is like a gentle wind that blows the clouds away, leaving a clear blue sky. The power of this single thought is in its repetition, which continually breaks the surface of attention to the exclusion of all other thoughts. The restrictive meditation process asks that you close your mind to external sensations and all outside stimulation and then direct the focus of your thoughts inward. In most cases, exclusive meditation is practiced with the eyes closed to prevent visual distractions.

There are five techniques that can help bring your attention to a single focused thought:

1. *Mental repetition:* Mental repetition is a thought that is consistently repeated. This thought is contained in a *mantra,* or a one-syllable word, such as "om," "one," "peace," or "love", that is repeated silently with the exhalation of each breath.

2. *Visual concentration:* Visual concentration involves staring at an object or image. Common visual images include a candle flame, a flower, a seashell, a picturesque scene, or a mandala.

3. *Repeated sounds:* Listening to repetitive sounds, such as a beating drum, chimes, bells, Gregorian chants, the rush of a waterfall, the sound of gentle ocean waves, rolling thunder, or some types of instrumental music can help you focus on a single thought.

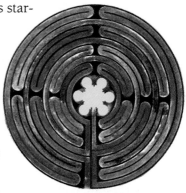

A mandala is a circle-shaped object, usually divided into quarters with intense color, intricate design, and beautifully detailed art.

4. *Physical repetitive motion:* Repetitive motion, such as breathing and some forms of rhythmic aerobic exercise (e.g., running, swimming, or walking), can produce a meditative state (the runner's high).

5. *Repeated tactile motion:* Holding and manipulating a small object such as a tumble stone, a seashell, or a string of beads can also help bring the mind to one thought.

Inclusive Meditation: Inclusive meditation is also referred to as "access meditation," "insightful meditation," or "mindfulness." Inclusive meditation appears to be very similar to *free association,* which lets your mind wander aimlessly. During inclusive meditation, your mind is free to accept all thoughts from both its conscious and unconscious mind. There is one condition, however. All thoughts that enter consciousness must do so objectively and without judgment or emotional attachment. This process is called *detached observation.* In effect, your mind becomes a movie screen with thoughts projected as images, and you observe without judgment or analysis. Ideally, by separating yourself from your emotions, you dissolve the walls of your ego temporarily, making you more open to ideas that can help you resolve issues in your life. In this type of meditation, the eyes are usually open, although you can close your eyes if you prefer.

The Relaxation Response

In his book *The Relaxation Response,* Dr. Herbert Benson describes how to meditate in four basic steps, creating a sense of calm and tranquillity. You will need a quiet environment, a comfortable position, a mental device, and a passive attitude.

1. *A quiet environment:* A quiet environment can be any place where you can relax without distractions such as ringing phones, doorbells, blaring televisions or radios, or outside street noise. You might find that you need to balance the quiet with white (background) noise, perhaps some soft instrumental music.

2. *A comfortable position:* Eastern philosophy suggests that to relax the mind, you must first relax the body. You should be in a comfortable position with your back straight. You should be relaxed, with no sense of muscular tension. If you feel as though you might fall asleep, sit up to meditate.

3. *A mental device:* A mental device is any method that is used to replace all other thoughts. It is a focal point to direct all attention. A mental device can include the repetition of a mantra, diaphragmatic breathing, or a Zen koan (an unanswerable question such as "What is the sound of one hand clapping?"). You might wish to combine a repetitive mantra with diaphragmatic breathing as a mental device.

4. *A passive attitude:* A passive attitude means that you are receptive, ready, and willing to relax. A passive attitude also includes a state of physical calmness. If your body is tense when you try to meditate, then the session will not be effective. In the words of Dr. Benson, "A passive attitude allows the meditative process to begin."

In today's high-tech age, you seldom experience real silence for any length of time. Because messages and information continually bombard you, your mind ends up getting choked. To keep your sanity, your mind needs to unload these thoughts. Regularly scheduled times of solitude can help you cleanse your cluttered mind.

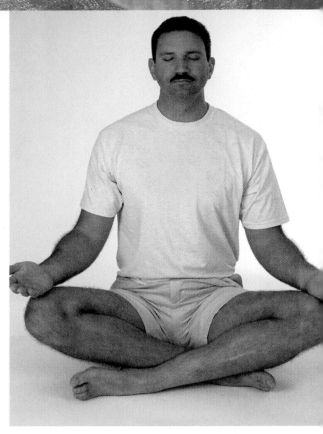

The best way to meditate is to find one place you can call your own where you can minimize distractions.

Mental Imagery

Close your eyes for a moment and imagine yourself at the ocean's shore. Listen to the gentle rolling waves. See the clear, aqua-blue water break as it approaches. Feel the white sand between your toes, the warm sun in your hair, and the soft wind as it caresses your face and continues on to sway the branches of a royal palm tree behind you. The salt air fills your lungs, and as you exhale, you feel completely relaxed. Imagination is a powerful gift. When Einstein said that imagination was more powerful than knowledge, he meant that the wealth of knowledge is grounded in the depths of human imagination. Sometimes, your imagination can distort problems, making mountains out of molehills. Yet your imagination can also serve as a tremendous defense against the effects of stress by transporting you to places of peace, relaxation, and restoration.

> **Imagination is more powerful than knowledge.**
> Albert Einstein

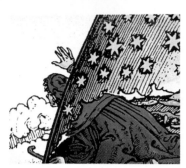

Using the power of your imagination means looking beyond the normal view of conscious thought.

A tranquil scene such as this is often used to promote relaxation.

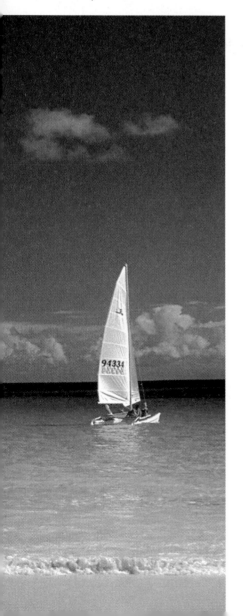

In simple terms, mental imagery is when you intentionally daydream. Mental imagery lets you make a motion picture. You take several active roles: the *producer,* who selects the sets and scenery; the *director,* who organizes the sensory cues; the *actor,* who feels and plays the part; and the *audience,* who experiences the effects of this production. These four roles are equally important in making the image as powerful as possible. With practice, you will enhance your skills in all these roles. You might find that mental imagery can be very enjoyable.

Mental imagery lets you access the powers of the conscious and unconscious minds to create a pictorial panorama that suggests calmness and tranquillity. It is also now used as a healing tool to restore health to body organs that are caught in a state of dysfunction and disease (such as cancer) and imagining those organs in a healthy state. The skill of mental imagery involves the creation of images, scenes, or impressions by engaging your imagination of your body's physical senses of sight, sound feel, smell, and even taste for a pleasurable mental sensation, such as going to the beach. In the case of a symbolic image, it could be the image of mending a broken bone.

Tranquil Natural Scenes

Natural settings are often selected to promote relaxation because nature is intrinsically calming to the human spirit. This is one reason why people vacation in the mountains or oceanside to escape the stresses of the home or work environment. Images such as a tropical island beach, a mountain vista, or a path through an evergreen forest are commonly used. Once created, these natural scenes, full of vivid color, fresh air, natural sounds and elements of nature, allow you to put your collective thoughts in true perspective. The effect of these natural scenes, like that of the real ones they imitate, can be to shrink perceptions and problems down to a manageable size, in proportion to the rest of the natural world. In essence, these tranquil images turn distorted perceptions back to manageable thoughts. And although the visualization of these scenes will not make personal problems go away, they do appear to help shrink troubles to a tolerable size. More important, with the repeated practice of visualization, heart rate and blood pressure begin to decrease, indicating a sense of calmness.

Of all the natural settings that are used to promote relaxation, the most common are those that include water, such as ocean beaches, mountain lakes, or waterfalls and streams. However, any scene that you think is relaxing can have the same effect. The power of this type of imagery is to use not just the imagination of the visual sense, but those of the other body senses as well. Seeing the image, hearing the sounds, smelling the fragrances or freshness of the air, sensing the air temperature, and feeling the wind and the sun on your skin all combine to create a powerful effect. By using all aspects of your imagination, you go from being a passive observer to an active participant in your own image. Furthermore, by acknowledging all sensations, you experience firsthand the calming effects of this technique rather than being an outside observer.

Body Position

Mental imagery, like diaphragmatic breathing, can be done almost anywhere. Simply close your eyes and tune out your current surroundings, allowing your imagination to create an image of peace and tranquillity. You can do this sitting or lying down.

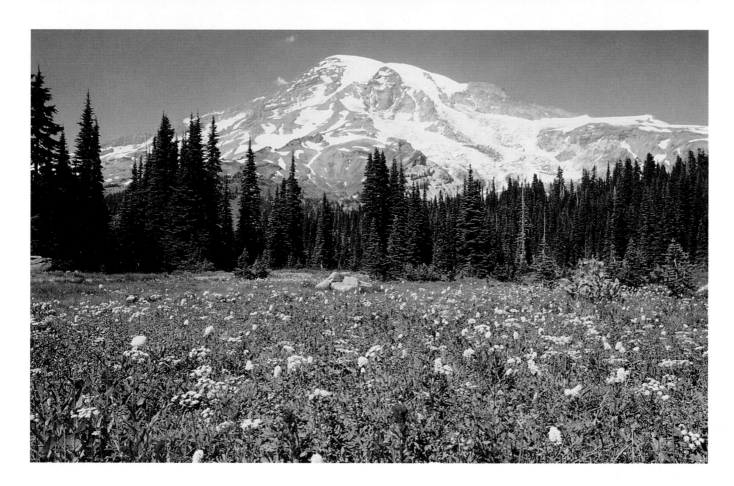

Concentration and Attitude

As with other relaxation techniques, mental imagery requires thorough concentration. Start with short periods (5 minutes) and allow your powers of concentration to build. Focus your attention toward the vividness of colors, shapes, textures, sounds, noises, silence, smells, and the entire feel of the environment you have created. If your mind begins to wander away from this scene, try to steer your attention back to the details of the image. Although it is best to learn mental imagery in a quiet environment, once you are proficient, you can use this technique in any situation in which you need to briefly close your eyes to escape momentarily and regain some composure (e.g., in the dentist's chair or on your lunch break). In terms of healing images such as cancerous tumors or broken bones, it is the experience of Doctors Bernie Siegel, Joan Borysenko, and Carl Simonton that the *belief* and *intention* in the power of the image are as important as the image itself.

Visual Themes

Your choice of mental images is unlimited. You can begin by deciding on the purpose of your visualization. Is it a momentary escape to clear your thoughts, or is the vision a healing image to rejuvenate your body and restore it to health? Once you decide, tailor your image to suit your needs, then close your eyes and go with it.

The purpose of relaxation techniques is to return the body to a state of homeostasis. Relaxation techniques work on one or more of the five senses to deactivate the stress response and reverse the body's adaptation to stress. Relaxation techniques go one step further to promote a deep sense of calm throughout the body, thereby promoting a greater sense of health and well-being.

stress | strategies

Exercise ①
Breathing Clouds

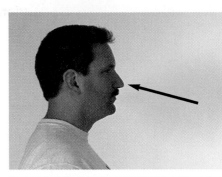

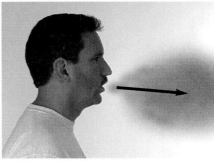

Diaphragmatic breathing can be traced back to India, with the practice of yoga, and Japan, with the practice of Zen meditation. It was introduced as a cleansing process for both the mind and body. To begin, close your eyes and focus all your attention on your breathing. Visualize the air that you take into your lungs as being clear, pure, and energized with the power to cleanse and heal your body. As you breathe in this clear, pure air, visualize and feel the air enter your nose (or mouth) and travel up through the sinus cavity to the top of your head and then continue down your spine and circulate throughout your lower stomach area. Now, as you exhale, visualize that the air leaving your body is dark air: a cloudy smoke that symbolizes all the stressors, frustrations, and toxins roaming throughout your mind and body. With each breath, allow the clean, pure air to enter, circulate, and rejuvenate your body. Let the exhaled dark air help to rid your body of its stress and tension. Repeat this breathing cycle for 5 to 10 minutes. Notice how your body releases stress and tension. You might also find that the color of the air exhaled changes from black to gray or off-white in a symbolic vision of complete relaxation.

Exercise ②
Relaxing Your Muscles

In this exercise, begin with the muscles of the face and contract the muscles for 5 seconds at three degrees of tension—100%, 50%, and 5%. Release and pause for about 45 seconds between each contraction. When you complete one muscle group, move to the next, starting with those in your face and working down to your feet.

Muscle group	100% Contraction	Release!	50% Contraction	Release!	5% Contraction	Release!
1. Face:	5 sec	45 sec	5 sec	45 sec	5 sec	45 sec
2. Jaws:	5 sec	45 sec	5 sec	45 sec	5 sec	45 sec
3. Neck:	5 sec	45 sec	5 sec	45 sec	5 sec	45 sec
4. Shoulders:	5 sec	45 sec	5 sec	45 sec	5 sec	45 sec
5. Upper chest:	5 sec	45 sec	5 sec	45 sec	5 sec	45 sec
6. Hands and forearms:	5 sec	45 sec	5 sec	45 sec	5 sec	45 sec
7. Abdominals:	5 sec	45 sec	5 sec	45 sec	5 sec	45 sec
8. Lower back:	5 sec	45 sec	5 sec	45 sec	5 sec	45 sec
9. Buttocks:	5 sec	45 sec	5 sec	45 sec	5 sec	45 sec
10. Thighs:	5 sec	45 sec	5 sec	45 sec	5 sec	45 sec
11. Calves:	5 sec	45 sec	5 sec	45 sec	5 sec	45 sec
12. Feet:	5 sec	45 sec	5 sec	45 sec	5 sec	45 sec

Exercise ③
Trying Autogenic Training

Take a slow, deep breath and feel the sense of relaxation throughout your body as you exhale. Make each breath even slower and deeper than the last. As you breathe, repeat these simple phrases to yourself:

Phase 1: Heaviness
- "My arms and hands feel heavy."
- "My legs and feet feel heavy."
- "My arms and legs feel heavy."

Phase 2: Warmth
- "My arms and hands feel warm."
- "My legs and feet feel warm."
- "My arms and legs feel warm."

Phase 3: Heart
- "My heart is calm and relaxed."
- "My heartbeat is slow and relaxed."

Phase 4: Breathing
- "My breathing is slow and relaxed."
- "My breathing is calm and comfortable."
- "My entire body is calm and relaxed."

Exercise ④
Making Exercise Work for You

To make sure that you are exercising at the right intensity for cardiovascular endurance, you should reach a target zone of 65% to 80% of your maximal capacity. Most people exercise at 75% capacity; however, if you are out of condition, you should see a physician first and start at a lower intensity. To calculate your target heart rate, use the formula shown. When you begin your exercise program, periodically check your heart rate to determine whether you are hitting your target. If you find that you are above your target heart rate, you are working too hard and should slow down a bit.

Maximal heart rate

220 (a constant value used by everyone)

− _____ age (fill in your age here)

= _____ (predicted maximal heart rate)

− _____ (subtract your resting heart rate here. You can determine your resting heart rate by taking your pulse for 60 seconds.)

x 0.75 (multiply 75% intensity of work load)

= _____ (heart rate reserve)

+ _____ (add back your resting heart rate)

* = _____ (your target heart rate)
  * You can divide this number by 6 for a 10-second count to make it easier when monitoring your heart rate during exercise.

_____ (divide by 6 for a 10-second count)

What is your preferred type of exercise?

_____

What time of day is best for you to exercise?

_____

What three days are best for you to exercise?

_____

Exercise ⑤
Looking at Eating

The association between nutrition and stress is a very important one. The following questions are provided for you to increase your awareness about the kinds of foods you eat and the stress behaviors associated with eating.

1. Do you regularly consume caffeine?   YES   NO

2. Please list the foods you ingest that contain caffeine and the estimated amounts that you consume (coffee, tea, sodas, chocolate, etc.).

   Types of food with caffeine   **Amount per day**

   1.

   2.

   3.

   4.

   5.

   6.

3. Do you take vitamin supplements?   YES   NO

   If so, what kind?_____ Are they bioavailable?   YES   NO

4. Do you frequently (every meal) use table salt   YES   NO

5. Do you eat one or more meals daily that are prepared outside the home?   YES   NO

6. Do you consume junk food (from vending machines, for example) regularly?   YES   NO

7. Do you eat cereals with sugar in them?   YES   NO

8. Do you drink a lot of soft drinks (sodas, pop)?   YES   NO

9. When you get stressed, do you tend to eat more?   YES   NO

10. When you are angry, do you tend to snack more?   YES   NO

11. Do you eat a wide variety of vegetables and fruits every day?   YES   NO

12. Do you eat foods such as fish and nuts that contain omega 3 and 6 (essential oils)?   YES   NO

13. Do you eat fats at each meal?   YES   NO

14. Please describe any of your eating habits that you associate with a stressed lifestyle.

   _____

   _____

   _____

   _____

   _____

15. On the basis of your answers to this assessment, how would you rate your stress eating habits?

   Awful   Poor   Fair   Good   Excellent

16. What is one way to change your eating behaviors to promote good nutrition?

Exercise ⑥
Relaxing to Music

1. Do you listen to music to relax?   YES   NO

2. What types of music do you like to listen to? Check all those that apply.

Classical _____   Jazz _____

Acoustic _____   Environmental _____

New age _____   Rock and roll _____

Blues _____   Reggae _____

Rap _____   Other _____

3. Of the categories listed above, distinguish between those you find energizing
and those you find calming.

ENERGIZING	CALMING
1.	1.
2.	2.
3.	3.
4.	4.
5.	5.

4. Who are your favorite music artists for calming music? Who are your favorite music artists
for energizing music? List them below.

CALMING	ENERGIZING
1.	1.
2.	2.
3.	3.
4.	4.
5.	5.

5. Do you play a musical instrument?   YES   NO

If so, which one(s)?

_____

6. On a scale of 1 (low) to 10 (high) how would you rate music as a relaxor? _____

7. On a scale of 1 (low) to 10 (high) how often do you use music as a means to relax? _____

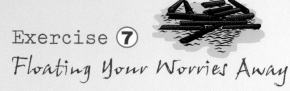

Exercise ⑦
Floating Your Worries Away

Close your eyes and imagine that you are sitting on a large rock by a river. As you look up the river, you see a logjam. You notice that the jam is beginning to slowly break up. One by one, each log is freed and swiftly moves through the currents traveling downstream. As you see each log, place a thought on it and then watch it move out of sight. Take a slow, deep breath and watch the next log approach. Once again let this log carry another thought out of sight. Continue to free all the logs from the logjam until your mind seems completely free of thoughts.

- When you do this exercise, sit comfortably in a chair or on the floor or lie down, keeping your spine aligned from your head to your hips.

- Observe your breathing by making each breath comfortably deep and relaxed.

- Use the log image as a repetitive mantra to help clear your mind of all thoughts.

- Initially, spend about 5 minutes on this exercise. Add more time as your comfort level increases.

Exercise ⑧
Rising Above Your Burdens

Close your eyes and imagine yourself in the basket of a hot air balloon. Firmly on the ground, the balloon is anchored by several sandbags. Picture each sandbag as some problem that weighs you down and that you wish to let go of.

One by one, release each sandbag. Slowly, let yourself begin to get lighter and lighter. Imagine the balloon lifting off the ground. As you slowly rise up into the sky, feel yourself become lighter and lighter.

Exercise ⑨
Creating Mental Images to Relax

When people think of peaceful scenes, they usually think of a natural setting. The best scenes seem to be far away from the hustle and bustle of the everyday world, a retreat to nurture the soul. Use your imagination to create some mental images that you think are examples of peaceful retreats. Describe in full detail five mental images or peaceful relaxing scenes where you would like to escape momentarily. Use all your senses to place yourself at each scene. Be as elaborate as you can with the description so that it will remain vivid in your memory.

1.

2.

3.

4.

5.

A Healthier Lifestyle

Chapter 5

Soon after his father died of a heart attack, Dave decided to get a physical exam, just to be on the safe side. Dave learned that he, too, at the age of 33, had several coronary risk factors.

Up to this point, he had thought he was immune to coronary heart disease—or any disease, for that matter. Although Dave dealt with death on a daily basis, his father's death hit too close to home. Dave began to examine some aspects of his own life. As a result, he changed some priorities, let some attitudes fall by the wayside, and gradually adopted some new behaviors. As Dave explained, he hasn't changed so much as he has evolved.

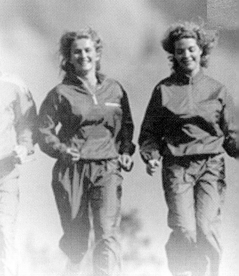

The Big Picture

Life, in all its complexity, is a mixture of emotional highs and lows, easy and difficult situations, and good and bad experiences. Quite simply, stress is a part of life. But it doesn't have to be the focus of our lives. Unfortunately, there are no quick fixes for everyday problems or work-related tensions. You do have invaluable inner resources, more commonly known as "muscles of the soul." These include, but are not limited to, patience, confidence, intuition, creativity, a sense of humor, courage, optimism, compassion, faith, and self-reliance. Anyone who has emerged from a difficult situation gracefully, without claiming victimization, will describe the skillful use of one or more of these muscles of the soul.

To deal with stress effectively, you must truly learn to cultivate your inner resources. In an effort to understand stress, experts have looked at the physical, psychological, social, environmental, and spiritual aspects and have come to the conclusion that work must begin *within* each individual to make the transition from stress-induced behaviors toward a stress-reduced lifestyle. As an EMS professional, you are more accustomed to taking care of others before you take care of yourself. Good stress management skills require a balancing act of honoring your own well-being (in mind, body, and spirit) just as you honor those you are called to assist.

By knowing yourself, examining your values, and working toward a fulfilling purpose in life, you can gain a better perspective on yourself, find a sense of balance in your day-to-day activities, and see how you fit comfortably into the bigger picture of life.

Focusing on yourself in this day and age is not easy. Distractions can block the process of nurturing the health of the human spirit. Making the time to nurture your own needs is not a selfish act. On the contrary, it is quite necessary. If you don't do so, you will soon have little or nothing to give others in need.

The winds of grace are blowing perpetually, we only need raise our sails.

Sri Ramakrishna

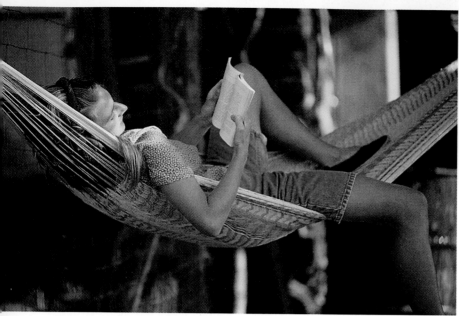

Making time for yourself to become centered and grounded is not a selfish act; it is essential for your own well-being.

Unbalanced, you become a bull's-eye target for everyday stressors.

The act of turning inward is often called the "centering process," in which you allocate some personal quiet time to sit alone each day, collecting and reflecting on your thoughts and feelings. Another person's death can act as a catalyst for this thought process, but it doesn't have to be, nor should it be, the only time for reflection. The fundamental purpose of coping and relaxation techniques is to create the opportunity for the centering process to occur, so that homeostasis of mind, body, and spirit is achieved. Once you become aware of the potential of your inner resources, you can tap them during stressful moments (e.g., frustrations with poor system designs, conflicts with various agencies, or working with an inexperienced partner). Like the deep roots of a tree, these inner resources help to keep you from being knocked over by the winds of change; however, these resources tend to manifest themselves professionally and/or personally. Psychologist Abraham Maslow called these inner resources "self-actualization traits." Through them, you can learn to consciously move beyond the mundane and chaotic parts of life to appreciate life's real beauty and perceive the "big picture." A healthy life *creates a balance* between the time dedicated to professional work and the time spent on personal needs. Achieving this balance might be challenging, but it's not impossible.

Purpose in Life

The answers to the meaning of your life come from a continual soul-searching process, not an outside source.

Medical experts conducting a study in the early 1990s in Massachusetts were baffled when they discovered that many first-time heart attack patients showed few of the known risk factors associated with heart disease. The most common characteristic is now reported to be job dissatisfaction. Many experts equate job dissatisfaction with a lack of meaning in life. This observance correlates highly with the fact that more heart attacks occur on Monday morning between 8:00 A.M. and 10:00 A.M. than at any other time during the week, a phenomenon called "Black Monday." Though much more difficult to measure than elevated cholesterol or blood pressure levels, a meaningful purpose in life is now thought to be a critical factor in the stability of your health. Establishing (or reestablishing) and evaluating your purpose in life also involves dedicating time to center and ground yourself. The coping and relaxation techniques in this book can help assist you in this process.

Letting Go of Stress: How to Maintain a Healthy Lifestyle

Most work-related stressors are based on the issue of control or the illusion of control. Think about how much time and personal energy you expend trying to

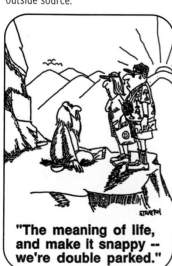

"The meaning of life, and make it snappy -- we're double parked."

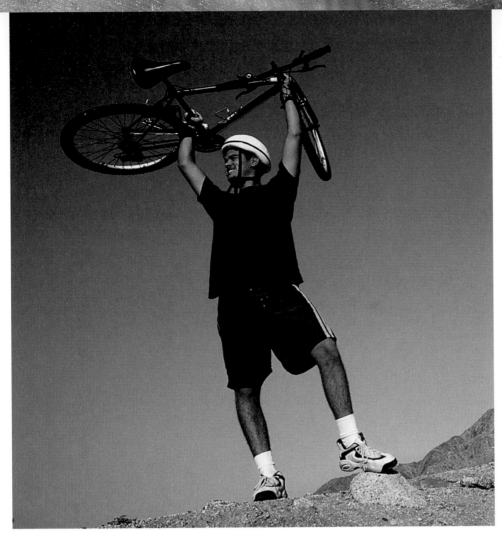

Achieving a goal or life purpose is one of the many ways to nurture the health of the human body.

influence and manipulate things over which you have no control. When you let go of stress, you focus on and empower yourself rather than trying to control events or people within your environment over which you have no control. It might take some effort, but you can learn to let go of stress.

Creating a personal stress management program is a very individual undertaking because no two people are alike. Several suggestions can help you find the path of least resistance, making your life journey less troublesome and more enjoyable.

1. *Respond* rather than react to situations that you find upsetting or a violation of your rights as an individual.
2. *Refine your expectations* and build a healthy tolerance toward situations that often disturb your inner balance.
3. *Give yourself positive feedback* through daily affirmations that validate your own self-esteem and worthiness. This practice might seem awkward at first, but give it a try and stick with it.
4. *Exercise regularly* to burn off any residual stress hormones that may be circulating in your body from a stressful day on the job. When your motivation is low, remember that walking is a great form of exercise.
5. *Incorporate some humor and mirth* into your daily routine to balance your scale of emotions. Gallows humor is great, but it's not the only kind of humor. Expand your humor repertoire to include other kinds of humor such as irony, slapstick, quick wit, and parody. Remember, avoid sarcasm.

6. *Nurture the connectedness* of the people in your circle of co-workers, friends, and family. If you feel that you lack support in your personal network, find the time to meet new people with similar interests in a sport, hobby, or support group and build new relationships that provide a buffer from daily stressors.

7. *Diversify your interests and activities* so that your whole identity is not wrapped up in your career or paycheck. This will not only make a bad day on the job more tolerable, it can actually improve your attitude about routine duties as well.

8. *Learn to recognize and become comfortable with all your emotions* and learn to express them creatively and productively.

9. *Exercise your creativity* and use this talent as well as other inner resources to relieve stress on the job and at home.

10. *Learn to resolve issues and concerns with others* when they arise, through peaceful and diplomatic confrontation rather than avoidance.

11. *Take short breaks in the course of each working day* to relax and give your body a chance to return to a normal resting state of homeostasis. You can accomplish this by spending 3 to 5 minutes doing breathing exercises, mental imagery, progressive muscular relaxation, or autogenic training.

12. *Take personal time for yourself every day* without feeling guilty. Take a few moments at the start or end of each day to sit quietly and meditate (center) or reflect on who you are and where you are going in your life. Start with as little as 5 minutes and build up from there.

Ultimately you must take responsibility for your own health. As a member of the health care industry, serving others must be balanced with taking care of yourself. Balance is the key to life!

 road to relaxation

Success

To laugh often and love much

To win the respect of intelligent persons and the affection of children

To earn the approval of honest critics and endure the betrayal of false friends

To appreciate beauty

To find the best in others

To give of oneself without the slightest thought of return

To have accomplished a task, whether by a healthy child, a rescued soul, a garden patch, or a redeemed social connection

To have played and laughed with enthusiasm and sung with exultation

To know that even one life has breathed easier because you have lived.

Anonymous

stress strategies

Exercise ①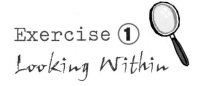
Looking Within

These attributes or inner resources are considered important tools to deal effectively with stress. Rate your sense of these qualities in yourself (0 = poor, 10 = excellent).

Attribute	Poor								Excellent	
Patience	1	2	3	4	5	6	7	8	9	10
Intuition	1	2	3	4	5	6	7	8	9	10
Creativity	1	2	3	4	5	6	7	8	9	10
Sense of humor	1	2	3	4	5	6	7	8	9	10
Confidence	1	2	3	4	5	6	7	8	9	10
Optimism	1	2	3	4	5	6	7	8	9	10
Compassion	1	2	3	4	5	6	7	8	9	10
Faith	1	2	3	4	5	6	7	8	9	10
Self-reliance	1	2	3	4	5	6	7	8	9	10

Spend a few minutes pondering these questions and then write down your thoughts

1. How well do you really know yourself at this point in time? What is your health philosophy and do you really practice it? How have your beliefs, attitudes, and opinions changed from just 5 years ago?

2. What aspects in life do you really value? What are the things that are most important in your life? Do you spend time living your values? Are some values in conflict with each other?

3. Where are you headed with your life? How would you define your life purpose at this time? Are you making progress toward it or do you seem to be in a period of stagnation?

4. What have you learned from your past experiences and how can you use these lessons to guide your life journey?

References and Resources

You might find that many topics in this workbook merit more attention. The following books can provide more information on the topics of mental, physical, emotional, and spiritual well-being.

Adams, K., *Journal to the Self.* New York: Warner Books, 1990.

Archteberg, J., *Imagery and Healing: Shamanism and Modern Medicine.* Boston: Shambhala Publications, 1985.

Beattie, M., *Codependent No More.* New York: Hazelton/Harper Press, 1987.

Beattie, M., *Beyond Codependence.* New York: Hazelton/Harper Press, 1989.

Benson, H., *The Relaxation Response.* New York: Morrow Press, 1975.

Borysenko, J., *Minding the Body, Mending the Mind.* New York: Bantam, 1984.

Borysenko, J., *Fire in the Soul: A New Psychology of Spiritual Optimism.* New York: Warner Books, 1993.

Buscaglia, L., *Love.* New York: Fawcett Crest, 1972.

Buscaglia, L., *Living, Loving and Learning.* New York: Fawcett Books, 1982.

Capacchione, L., *The Creative Journal: The Art of Finding Yourself.* Athens, GA: Swallow Press, 1979.

Casey, K., and Vanceburg, M., *The Promise of a New Day.* New York: Harper & Row, 1983.

Chopra, D., *Quantum Healing.* New York: Bantam Books, 1989.

Cooper, K., *The Aerobics Program for Total Well-Being.* New York: Bantam Books, 1983.

Covey, S., *The Seven Habits of Highly Effective People.* New York: Fireside/Simon and Schuster, 1989.

Covey, S., *First Things First.* New York: Simon and Schuster, 1994.

Dossey, L., *Recovery of the Soul.* New York: Bantam Books, 1989.

Dossey, L., *Healing Words: The Power of Prayer and the Practice of Medicine.* San Francisco: Harper Collins, 1993.

Dyer, W., *Your Erroneous Zones.* New York: Avon Books, 1976.

Fanning, P., *Visualization for Change.* Oakland, CA: New Harbinger Publications, 1976.

Foster, S., and Little, M., *The Book of the Vision Quest.* New York: Prentice Hall, 1988.

Frankl, V., *Man's Search for Meaning.* New York: Pocket Books, 1984.

Goleman, D., *Emotional Intelligence*. New York: Bantam Books, 1996.

Jacobson, E., *You Must Relax*. New York: McGraw Hill, 1978.

Jampolski, G., *Love Is Letting Go of Fear*. Berkeley, CA: Celestial Arts, 1979.

Klein, A. *The Healing Power of Humor*. Los Angeles: Tarcher Press, 1989.

Kübler-Ross, E., *Death, the Final Stage of Growth*. New York: Touchstone Books, 1987.

Lerner, Harriet, *The Dance of Anger*. New York: Harper and Row, 1985.

Lindbergh, A. M., *Gift from the Sea*. New York: Vintage Books, 1978.

Moyers, Bill, *Healing and the Mind*. New York: Anchor Press, 1993.

Peck, M. Scott, *The Road Less Traveled*. New York: Touchstone Press, 1978.

Peter, L., and Dana, B., *The Laughter Prescription*. New York: Ballantine Press, 1982.

Robbins, A., *Awakening the Giant Within*. New York: Simon and Schuster, 1992.

Schaef, A. W., *Co-Dependence: Misunderstood, Mistreated*. New York: Harper and Row, 1986.

Seaward, B.L., *Stand Like Mountain, Flow Like Water: Reflections on Stress and Human Spirituality*. Deerfield Beach, FL: Health Communications Inc., 1997.

Seaward, B.L., *Managing Stress: Principles and Strategies for Health and Wellbeing, Second Edition, WWW enhanced*. Sudbury, MA: Jones and Bartlett, 1999.

Seaward, B.L., *Stressed Is Desserts Spelled Backwards: Rising above Life's Challenges with Humor, Hope and Courage*. Berkeley, CA: Conari Press, 1999.

Seaward, B.L., *The Art of Calm : Relaxation Through the Five Senses*. Deerfield Beach, FL: Health Communications, Inc., 1999.

Siegel, B., *Love, Medicine and Miracles*. New York: Perennial Press, 1987.

Siegel, B., *Peace, Love, and Healing*. New York: Perennial Press, 1990.

Selye, H., *Stress without Distress*. New York: Signet Books, 1987.

Simonton, O.C., *Getting Well Again*. New York: Bantam Books, 1978.

von Oech, R., *A Whack in the Side of the Head*. New York: Warner Books, 1983.

von Oech, R., *A Kick in the Seat of the Pants*. New York: Perennial Library, 1986.

Weisinger, H., *The Anger Workout Book*. New York: Quill Books, 1985.

Photo Credits

Chapter 1
p. 2, Courtesy of the American Academy of Orthopaedic Surgeons; p.3, © Ziggy and Friends, Inc.; p. 5 bottom, © Tracy Mack, In the Dark Photography; p. 6 bottom, © John Mielcarek, 911 Pictures; p. 8 top, © Linda Gheen; p. 8 bottom courtesy of the American Academy of Orthopaedic Surgeons

Chapter 2
p. 13, © Michael Kowal, Custom Medical; p. 14, © Steve Spak, 911 Pictures; p. 16, © Sean O'Brien, Custom Medical; p. 20 top, Courtesy of the American Academy of Orthopaedic Surgeons; p. 20 bottom, © Ziggy and Friends, Inc.; p. 21 © Linda Gheen; p. 24, © Oscar Burriel, Photo Researchers

Chapter 3
p. 31, © Lowell Georgia, Photo Researchers Inc.; p. 32 top, Calvin and Hobbes copyright Watterson; p. 32 bottom, © Ziggy and Friends, Inc.; p. 35 top, left and right, The Far Side © 1990 Farworks, Inc.; p. 36 bottom, Courtesy of NASA; p. 42 bottom © Bob Daemmrich, The Image Works; p. 43, Calvin and Hobbes copyright Watterson

Chapter 4
p. 56 bottom, © Ziggy and Friends, Inc.; p. 64, CATHY copyright Cathy Guisewite

Chapter 5
p. 78 © Stratton

Charts/Illustrations
The charts on the following pages created by Studio Montage.

Chapter 1
p. 4

Chapter 3
p. 38, top; p. 40, top

Chapter 4
p. 63, top

Index

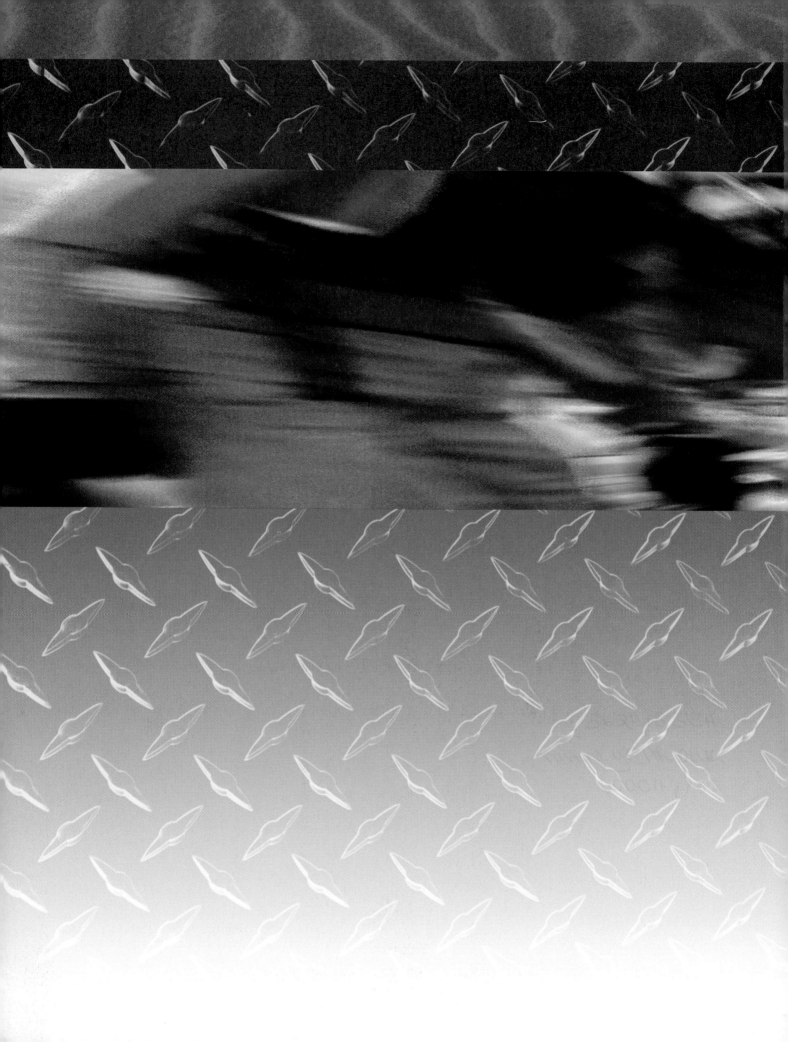

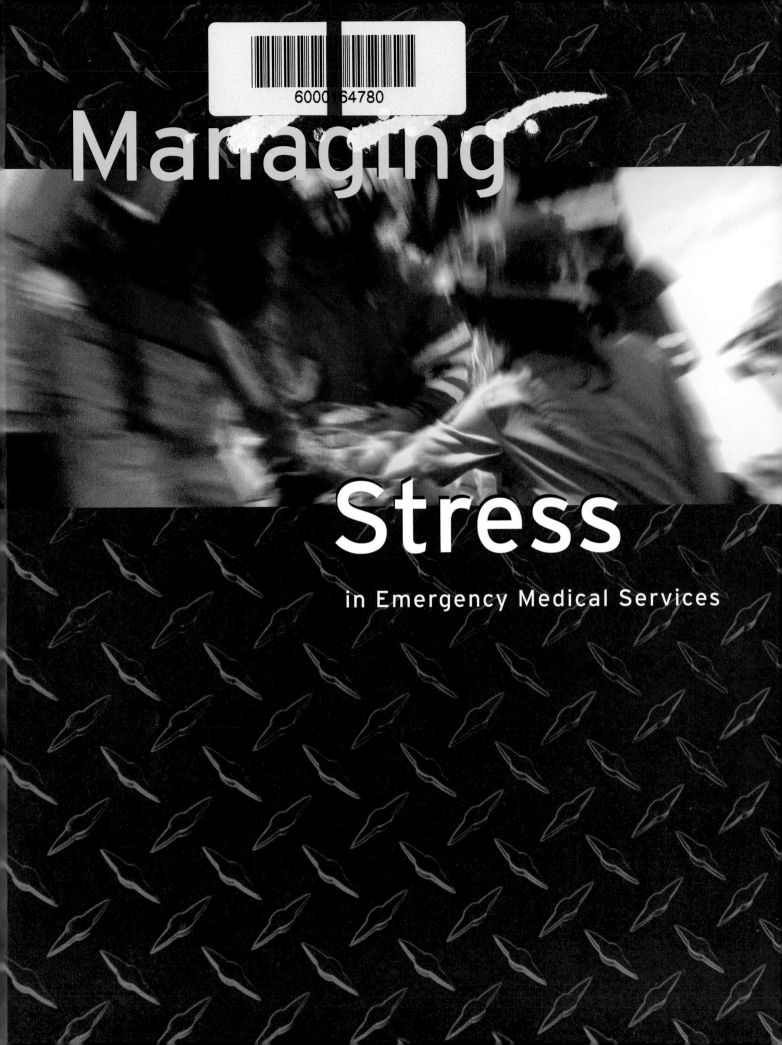

Managing

Stress

in Emergency Medical Services